THIRTY PLANTS
THAT CAN SAVE
YOUR LIFE!

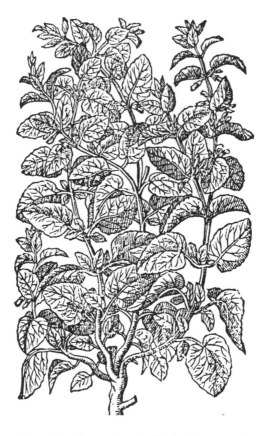

Most of the illustrations in this book are wood-
cuts from the 1633 edition of Gerard's *Herball*
as compiled by Thomas Johnson. In the 1600s
botanists routinely lent, borrowed, copied, and
stole woodblocks from each other. Many of the
images that appear in Gerard's volume had
appeared earlier in the *Rariorum plantarum
historia*, a 1601 botanical masterwork by Carolus
Clusius, the father of descriptive botany.

THIRTY PLANTS
THAT CAN SAVE
YOUR LIFE!

By DOUGLAS SCHAR

ELLIOTT & CLARK PUBLISHING
Washington, D.C.

DEDICATED TO MY GRANDMOTHER ARLENE WINKLER, MY MOTHER
JANICE SCHAR, AND MY PARTNER IN CRIME KATE CALDWELL.

Designed by Gibson Parsons Design
Edited by Elizabeth Brown Lockman

Second Printing 1995
Printed and bound in U.S.A.

Any inquiries should be directed to:
ELLIOTT & CLARK PUBLISHING
P.O. Box 21038
Washington, DC 20009-0538
Telephone (202) 387-9805

Library of Congress Cataloging-in-Publication Data
Schar, Douglas, 1964–
    Thirty plants that can save your life / Douglas Schar.
      p.   cm.
    ISBN 1-880216-09-4
    1. Herbs—Therapautic use. 2. Materia medica, Vegetable.
  I. Title.
  RM666.H33S33 1992
  615'.321—dc20   92-38634
                                  CIP

The author has based the material in this book on reliable historical and
scientific sources as well as upon his own personal experiences. Every
effort has been made to note potentially dangerous herbs and potencies.
The author, however, makes no guarantees as to the curative effect of any
herb or tonic in this book, and no reader should attempt to use any of the
information herein provided as treatment for any illness, weakness, or
disease without first consulting a physician. Pregnant women should
always consult first with a health-care professional before taking any
treatment.

CONTENTS

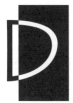id that title catch your eye? I wanted you to pick this book off the shelf because I have some important information I want you to know about: 30 plants that could literally save your life. I know, it sounds like an outrageous claim, but as you read a little further, I think you will agree.

For the most part, and I know there are exceptions, people's survival instinct runs pretty strong. This instinct is the part of your brain that emits messages such as: "there's an electrical storm outside, better not mow the grass right now," or "don't lean over the edge of the balcony." It's what I like to call the universal theme: our desire to live in safety and good health for as long as we possibly can. This same instinct directed you to pick up this book. Self-preservation has also fueled the human discovery process for thousands of years.

Up until very recently, human beings have looked to the plants of the jungles or the plains or the mountains to help them out, at least in the health department. No one knows exactly how this process started, how the first man or woman figured out that the plants growing in his or her very midst could strengthen the body. By the time the Bible was written, the use of plants as agents of health had developed into a complex body of knowledge. But research didn't stop at the biblical period. It continued for an additional 2,000 years.

The strange thing about this knowledge of health-boosting plants is that in the past 100 years—the span of a few generations—it has been almost entirely forgotten. What was once commonly known is now a coveted secret. Most of us don't include it in our health-preservation routines because we aren't even aware it exists. But it does. The information we all need to help make our lives longer and healthier is sitting in library stacks, waiting to be put to use. And practically no one is taking advantage of it.

Thirty Plants That Can Save Your Life is a manual designed to help you rediscover these discoveries lost. To do so, we need to have a starting point, and ours will be the top 30 plants used for staying well since time immemorial.

There are thousands of healing plants on our planet, more than enough to overwhelm even the most tireless and health-conscious researcher. With so many to choose from, let me explain how I selected these 30 plants. I went through several hundred herbals, or books about healing plants, from all over the world—Europe, Africa, Asia, you name the country—and every time a plant was mentioned as one boosting overall bodily health, I entered it into my computer.

I believe there is safety in numbers, and the plants I selected for this book are the ones that were cited most often worldwide for their health-preserving powers. For one reason or another, the global community came to the same conclusions about these same plants over and over again. The result of my selection process is a world consensus. These are the top 30 health-giving plants.

One point I would like to clear up right away concerns the accuracy and validity of the herbals I used to create my initial list. Obviously, if the original data was a crock of crap, then the more refined list of plants would merely be a more refined crock of crap. Are these herbals filled with useful information about plants that really can heal? Of course they are. Take a look at just a few of the plants included in this book and how long they have been in active medicinal use: licorice, 3,000 years; ginseng, 4,000 years; dates, 5,000 years.

Do you think people around the world would have used these plants day in and day out for such long periods of time if they did not, in fact, have some positive effects on the human body? Of course not. Anywhere you go, human consumers are a pain in the butt. If a consumer buys a product and it doesn't work, he or she either takes it back or doesn't buy it again.

Let's consider a hypothetical situation. You have a wicked case of the intestinal flu, you are losing it from both ends, and you wish that somebody would take you out behind the barn and finish the job. You send someone to the store to pick up medicine, you take it, and you are still as sick as a dog. The next time you have the flu, will you send someone out for the same product? Odds are you will try a new one instead. This scenario is true universally: people don't use medicines that don't work, at least not a second time. Folks have been buying ginseng for 4,000 years because it works. The plants in this book are powerful medicine, and they have stood the consumer test of time.

Although the majority of the plants we will be working with are also used to treat specific conditions, their most interesting attribute is their ability to preserve health in general and to keep the body from going bad. Western medicine is almost entirely consumed with treating illnesses, taking care of problems once they have already appeared. If you don't believe me, go to the doctor, say you want a prescription to avoid getting a cold this winter, and see what he or she has to offer. It won't be a lot. Western medicine doesn't have much in the way of prevention. The old herbals do.

Though the modern world is filled with psychological stresses, life for many of us just isn't as physically demanding as it was in days gone by. It used to be that practically everyone worked with his or her body. When most people farmed for a living, they needed to be as strong as possible during the planting and harvesting seasons, and they took herbs to make sure that this was the case. An interesting story along these lines comes from my father's side of the family. It seems that my great-grandfather up and died right before harvest time. His widow had several fields full of crops and a house full of kids—a bad combination. She couldn't afford to sit around and cry. Instead, she immediately married a man with a strong back, and my great-grandmother, her new husband, and the kids got the harvest to market on time.

From a time in world history when keeping well and strong was the best and only chance you and your family had of staying alive, a concept developed of what we would now call preventative medicine. In those days, the word assigned to the concept was *tonic*. Plants noted for their ability to keep the body fit were called tonic plants, and medicines produced from these plants were called tonics. Let's look at my copy of the *Century Dictionary*, printed in 1889, and see how it defines *tonic*: "In medicine, increasing the strength or the tone of the animal system; obviating the effects of weakness or debility, and restoring healthy functions; hence, bracing or invigorating to the mental or moral nature." I chose this dictionary because it was printed when people were still using tonics, taking them much the same way we take chemically synthesized vitamins. Every day after breakfast, everybody in the family got a tablespoon of Mom's recipe. You'd better believe that my grandmother's number-two man got one before he left the house every morning!

You may be wondering why these tonic plants and remedies fell from common use. There are a number of factors, but a major one was the general migration from the farm to the factory which took place in the United States between

World Wars I and II. As people moved from places with few doctors to places with many doctors, they began to rely on professionals rather than on family members for their health care. The plants they had once gathered freely in the woods and fields surrounding their homes were simply not available in the city. But newly manufactured chemical medications were, and our love affair with the tablet began.

I did a little survey among the doctors I came into contact with over the past year. When I casually asked them what they thought of the tonics and tonic plants which were so popular in the past century and all the centuries that preceded it, the standard response was: "Tonics were old wives' tales." You will note that I used the word "thought" instead of "knew" because I quickly found out that none of these esteemed physicians knew anything at all about tonics. None had ever used tonics, seen tonics, researched tonics. It's interesting that the doctors were so quick to say tonics had no value when they themselves had no knowledge of the topic. I point this out because most of us share the same attitude: we assume that tonics are of no value before any examination of the facts. Contempt prior to investigation is active stupidity. Back to my point that people don't use products that don't work, men and women living 100 years ago knew what our modern doctors do not. They made and took tonics regularly because when they did, they saw a real difference in the way that they felt.

Doctors' ignorance of tonic plants and formulas is a relatively new phenomenon, an offshoot of our shift from a primarily rural to an urban society. Before the turn of the century, the most successful physicians were those gifted in concocting tonic formulas to give to their patients. One doctor, a certain A. W. Chase, was so famous for his tonics, many of which featured herbs on our list of the top 30 plants, that he compiled them into a book entitled *Dr. Chase's Receipt Book and Household Physician, or Practical Knowledge for the People*. Published in 1892, his book sold hundreds and thousands of copies. Why? For the simple reason that Dr. Chase's formulas worked. When people mixed them up and took them, they felt better.

In time, the commercial making of tonics became a big business as people who dreamed up particularly good formulas took them to the public. Many of our modern drug companies were founded in the days of the tonic trade. Some companies produced the tonics themselves, and others sold the ingredients out of which home tonics were brewed. The W. E. Servall Company was such a concern. This statement comes from their 1917 catalogue:

Knowing that there is not a plant, herb, root, or bark found in nature's laboratory which does not possess its own special remedial value, it requires no flight of the imagination to realize that when a combination is made of such as act wholesomely upon any organ of the body, each in its different way, the combined result can but lead to that which we all desire most—HEALTH with all its attendant blessings.

The Servall Company suggested that people make their own tonics. Today we have no other choice if we want to enjoy the life-giving properties of the herbs that men, women, and children across the planet have used and trusted for thousands of years. The plants you will read about on the following pages are all tonic plants. When they are used judiciously, they can both refresh and invigorate the body. Correctly taken on a daily basis, these 30 plants can keep you healthy, and when you are healthy, you don't get sick.

This is an activity book. First we are going to do some background reading on the top tonic plants, including what specific conditions they treat, as we all have our pet illnesses, and it's good to know which herbs will take care of them. Then we are going to learn how to take these plants and make what I call the "Turbo Tonic," an incredible tonic that can keep you well. The herbs can be used separately or in combination, but as the Servall Company's catalogue states, "the combined result can but lead to that which we all desire most—HEALTH," and that's what we're aiming for here. I have also included several simpler, more specific tonic recipes for those of you with special concerns and a chapter on how to get or grow the plants you'll need. What are we waiting for? Let's jump right in and learn how to start saving our lives.

Dayle Scher

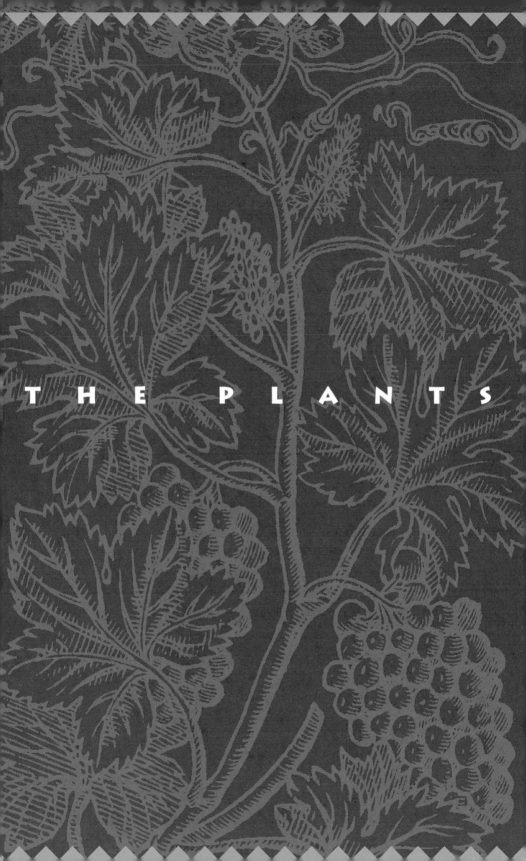

THE PLANTS

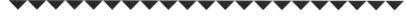

ANGELICA

Angelica archangelica

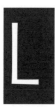et's start our meet-and-greet session with angelica, a plant the ancients thought was so heavenly that they named it after the angels. More than 50 varieties grow all over the globe, and each and every angelica has been recognized by its neighbors as having special powers in promoting good health.

What's more, all the angelicas are used for the same purpose regardless of where they are found: staying well.

Angelica belongs to one of the most magical families of plants on the planet, the umbelliferae family, named for the umbrella-shaped flower head of its members. These include carrots, parsnips, parsley, coriander, dill, chervil, celery, anise, cumin, and asafoetida, to mention a few. Although the umbelliferaes are noted worldwide for their medicinal touch, every family has its overachievers, and angelica soars above its relations in this department. There is a notion among herbalists past and present, one that I know to be true: for every disease nature makes, it also makes a plant that will cure it. Considering angelica's track record, it would seem that Mother Nature was killing a few birds with a single stone when she dreamed up this one.

Angelica looks like a carrot plant with one small exception. A carrot plant rarely reaches 12 inches in height; angelica can easily reach 10 feet. When you look at an angelica plant, you can actually see its power.

Chinese medicine uses nine angelica species. Collectively, these are known as *dang quei*, and the angelica of choice is *Angelica chinensis*. Dating to 400 B.C., angelica is one of the first recorded Chinese drugs, and it's still in common use today.

If ginseng is the main herb used in China as a male tonic, angelica is its female counterpart. Possessing a set of ovaries and a uterus is risky business, and was much more so in days gone by. The Chinese observed that women who took angelica on a daily basis conceived easily, didn't miscarry, delivered safely, and breezed through menopause with no problem. (Although during pregnancy, angelica should only be used under the care of a qualified herbalist.) And most importantly, women on angelica didn't suffer from the monthly visitor as badly as those not on angelica.

The Chinese also believe that women who take angelica maintain their youth far beyond its usual term. Consequently, they include it in all their major beauty

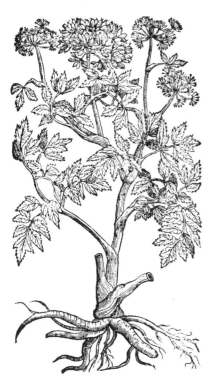

creams. This sounded like an old wives' tale to me until one day when I was buying some props (for my television show "Urban Gardener") at the Chinese herbalist's and an attractive woman walked in. We started talking about Chinese herbs and their efficacy, and she asked what I thought her age was. I said 35; she answered 72. She then pulled out pictures of her mother who could have passed for 55. The mother's real age was 91. What was the woman buying that day? Angelica.

But traditional Chinese use of the plant goes far beyond this. They take angelica to beef up every major organ, including the skin. How does this stand up to the scientific research process we all believe in so absolutely?

Chinese medicine uses angelica to treat people with overwrought nervous systems. More simply put, that's folks who edge on the neurotic, and science has proven that angelica is a mild sedative, just what the doctor ordered. *Dang quei* is also used to treat allergies and all their annoying symptoms. In the lab, allergic response suppression activity was observed with both oral and injected root extracts. Scientists have been linking allergies and arthritis in recent days, and angelica is also used for creaky joints. As the Chinese believe, it likewise has been proven to lower arterial pressure and prevent cancer.

One of the most important health claims from the Chinese countryside is that angelica, taken regularly, is plain good for you. In that it works on all major body parts, this claim seems quite reasonable. But more than that, chemicals contained in angelica kill bacteria, fungus, and viruses. As these little bad boys are the microbes that bring on colds and infections, knocking them out every day would indeed prevent illness. You really can't lose with angelica.

The European angelica, *Archangelica*, first appears in medical literature in the Middle Ages, smack dab during the years when the black plague swept through Europe's cities, leaving so few people alive to bury the dead that bodies were piled on the street corners. Legend holds that God saw what was happening on earth and sent the Archangel Michael to reveal the plant's healing power. Angelica had grown alongside European gardens for centuries, and for whatever reason, people started noticing it just at the time it could do the most good.

Once the Europeans discovered the plant's powers, they quickly started using it for all sorts of ills and weaknesses. In 1578, an herbalist by the name of Turner said of angelica, "It defends the heart against all poisons." The common thought in the 16th century was that angelica was a "counterbane," or cure-all, capable of counteracting whatever was wrong with you.

Gerard, an herbal scientist living during the turn of the 17th century, observed:

The root of garden angelica is a singular remedy against poison, and against the plague, and all infections taken by evil and corrupt air; if you do but take a piece of the root and hold in it your mouth, or chew the same between your teeth, it doth most certainly drive away the pestilential air, yeah, although that corrupt air have possessed the heart, yet it driveth it out again by urine and sweat.

Was Gerard all washed up? Absolutely not. Bacteria are, in fact, airborne, and like Chinese angelica, European angelica has been proven to kill bacteria and viruses.

Though the plant came to the fore during the plague years, it lingered on and found a number of uses in maintaining health. Like the Chinese, the Europeans used it for treating bronchial colds, circulation problems, muscle spasms, rheumatism, inflammation of the intestinal tract, indigestion, stomach cancer, water retention, tumors and sores that won't heal, insomnia, lack of energy, and debility.

In the Americas, the purple angelica, *Angelica purpoutrea*, was used both by the Native Americans and by the colonials who came and booted out the natives.

Native Americans used the root, leaves, and seeds of the purple angelica as a treatment par excellence for the stomach. They shared this information with the colonials, who certainly needed it, as the European intestinal tract wasn't accustomed to the local bacteria and viruses. The natives also used it as a general tonic, particularly against chronic illnesses such as cancer or colds that wouldn't go away. It seems to me that years ago when a person got a cold, it was gone in a week, not to resurface for another year. Today, we have these colds that can last for months, and this is exactly the situation Native Americans used angelica to clear up.

Around the globe, angelica is seen as what in modern lingo might be called an immunity plant. Though many of the health claims about it have been substantiated, many more have not yet been researched. However, all facts indicate that there is something special contained in this plant. That something may not ever be tacked down by science, but who cares? If it works, use it.

ANGELICA. Though it is good for both sexes, the Chinese hold it as a must for women. Here's how a female friend of mine recommends taking angelica. Boil one cup of angelica root in a quart of water for five minutes. After the mixture cools, pour it into an empty plastic water bottle and keep it in the fridge. Every once in a while, take a cooling swig. The bottle goes with her on bike rides and other exercise adventures. I like her habit so much that I've taken to doing the same thing.

For our tonic, the Chinese Angelica can be purchased at Chinese pharmacies, and the European can be had at most natural food stores. As with all produce, fresh is better, and you might want to put a row of angelica in your garden for a constant and ready supply. The European plants are available from most mail-order herb companies. Because the seeds don't remain viable long enough to survive shipping, one-year-old plants which will take root immediately in the garden are sent through the mail.

Angelica is actually a biennial, but you can trick it into being a perennial by not allowing it to go to seed. Once the plant produces seeds, angelica keels over and dies. However, if you cut the flower head off before it goes too far, the plant will spread instead, and what was once a single plant will become a clump and then a thicket of angelica.

The root is harvested on an as-needed basis—it stays good in the ground forever, so you can gather this ingredient whenever you want to make your tonic. The root, along with the stems and leaves, can also be collected and dried for tonic purposes.

ASTRAGALUS

Astragalus membranaceus

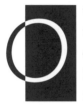ur next plant, astragalus, is grown almost exclusively in Asia, and in the aim of understanding its importance, I thought we would take a crash course in the Chinese medical system. As they say, when in Rome, don't run around speaking Greek. Though Westerners tend to think of Chinese medicine, or at least what they know of it—acupuncture, massage therapy, and the like—as something new, it is only new to us. When the Europeans were still wearing bear skins and bopping future dates over the head with clubs, the Chinese were scientifically studying plants and recording their findings. Their medical system is hundreds of years older than ours, and they have had a long time to work out the kinks. I bother pointing this out because most Westerners look at Chinese medicine a bit askance. When you realize how old the system is, you may not question it quite as much.

One of the oldest medical documents in China dates to somewhere between 200 and 100 B.C. Named the *Yellow Emperor's Inner Classic*, it forms the philosophical foundation for Chinese medicine. The book espouses proper diet, physical fitness, and the use of herbs to stay well. It may have taken us Westerners 2,100 years to figure this out, but at last we are starting to see what the writers of the *Yellow Emperor's Inner Classic* already knew.

One of the 13 questions the Yellow Emperor asks his doctors in this important piece of literature is why, unlike in days gone by, prayer is no longer sufficient to bring about health. The doctors respond that people are living hectic, unhealthy lives and that prayer is just not enough anymore. They insist that in the "modern" world (remember, this is 200 B.C.) folks have to do more to stay healthy. Sound familiar? This is precisely where we are today—we too have to do more to stay well.

The *Yellow Emperor's Inner Classic* views the human being as part of the natural world, subject to the same rules that apply to the other parts. If you don't water a plant, it withers and dies; if you don't water a man, he withers and dies. Disease happens when the body gets out of balance. We've all used phrases like "she worked herself to death" and "he drove himself crazy," and we all know what it's like to work so hard on a project for so long that you come down with a whopper of a cold when it's done. In essence, this first Chinese medical book establishes the same thought: if you live out of balance, you are going to get sick.

The important distinction between Chinese and Western medicine becomes

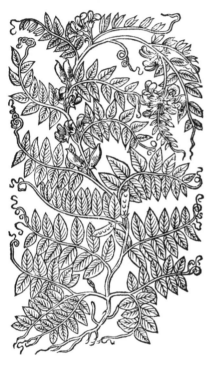

clear at this point. Chinese medicine is all about balancing the body so that you never get sick. Western medicine is all about picking up the pieces once the system has broken down.

Whereas the *Yellow Emperor's Inner Classic* is a statement of philosophy, another Chinese document, *The Divine Husbandman's Classic of the Materia Medica*, is the book that tells what to do, when to do it, and under what circumstances. Said to have been compiled in the first century A.D. and by a "divine husbandman" at that, the volume goes into the specifics of bringing the body into balance. It includes 252 plants, 45 minerals, and 67 animal substances that promote permanent health. Enter our next plant that could save your life.

Listed in *The Divine Husbandman's Classic* as a number-one health-keeping plant, astragalus, that body balancer extraordinaire, has been in continuous use for the past 2,000 years. I hate to pull rank, but our little Western pills have only been around for a century, and the doubter out there should probably take the cotton out of his or her ears at this point and put it in his or her mouth. Does astragalus work? Of course it does.

The astragalus that makes its way into the Chinese pharmacy is actually the root of the plant. The plant itself is a member of the highly helpful and healthful legume family, which also includes clover and licorice. Its scientific name, *Astragalus membranaceus*, or "the astragalus with lots of membranes," refers to the fact that the root is filled with them. They readily pull apart and shred into a million smaller pieces, rather like tissue paper. The roots used medicinally are harvested in several provinces, then shipped from those points to the rest of the country and the world.

In Chinese medicine, different herbs are said to enter the body through different paths: astragalus enters through the lung and spleen channels. As such, it is thought to act as a tonic for these organs. The common symptoms of someone in need of astragalus are chronic fatigue, lack of appetite, and chronic diarrhea, all said to be the body's way of telling the patient that his or her spleen isn't working well and needs a boost. Other physical problems for which astragalus is the treatment are: anorexia, arthritis, cancer, diabetes mellitus, high blood pressure, malaria, inflammation of the kidneys, painful urination, a prolapsed uterus, stomach, or anus, uterine bleeding and weakness, edema, water retention, skin ulcers that won't heal, fever, lack of stamina, and overall weakness.

Just for fun, let's check out some of these claims with the modern scientific community and see what they have learned about astragalus. The extracts of astragalus have been found to kill bacteria and lower blood sugar and blood pressure. Its blood-pressure lowering activity is said to be due to the gamma-aminobutyric acid contained within the plant. When it is injected into animals, they experience a drop in blood pressure apparently due to direct dilation of the blood vessels. This indicates that the plant would indeed be useful in treating someone with high blood pressure. Its ability to lower blood sugar explains its usefulness in treating diabetes.

Astragalus is one of the classic Chinese plants used to strengthen the respiratory tract and fight upper respiratory infections. Chemicals contained in the root have been found to strengthen the cells that make up the lungs. Its tonic effect combined with its antibacterial effect explain why astragalus is a good plant for someone with a lung infection.

ASTRAGALUS. The first time you buy this root at the herbalist's, you'll think that the person misunderstood your request and handed you tongue depressors! Never fear; the narrow, sliced sticks are what you're after. After visiting my sister's children—the original petri dishes of disease—I boil five or six astragalus slices in three cups of water. When the liquid is reduced to one cup, I drink it with a teaspoon of honey and hope for the best. Sometimes if my nephews have something really bad, like chicken pox, I chew on one of the sticks on the way over and one on the way home.

Kidneys are the organ that pumps the water out of your body, and what goes out with this water? Harmful toxins. Astragalus has a long-acting diuretic effect on humans which substantiates its use in treating swelling and water retention. In addition to getting the kidneys pumping, astragalus tones the organ itself.

In a bizarre experiment, the Chinese found that the stamina of mice given astragalus enemas and douches was much increased in swimming tests. The conclusion is that astragalus might likewise give the human body increased stamina, and who couldn't use that?

In yet another study, the Chinese found that mice fed astragalus for a number of days were able to protect themselves from absorbing a toxic chemical into their livers. This is saying that the body effectively eliminated the toxin—no small thing. In a world filled with environmental- and self-pollution, our livers have to work overtime, and a liver tonic is what everybody needs.

For practical, day-to-day use, astragalus increases the energy and builds resistance to disease. It acts as a tonic to the blood, lungs, kidneys, and spleen. The Chinese believe that it warms the blood and balances the energies in the internal organs. Remember, a balanced body is one that doesn't get sick, and that's our goal: staying well so that we don't waste our personal-leave days lying in front of the television.

Aside from being a tonic for the blood, lungs, kidneys, and spleen, astragalus also directs medicines into those parts of the body. It's what is known as an assisting herb. If you are having a problem with your lungs, astragalus will shoot the herb you are taking for it straight to the place it will do the most good.

Astragalus is the plant the Chinese recommend when you have used up all your vitality. It is not, of course, so powerful that you can continually abuse your body and never pay the piper, but when occasions of stress occur, astragalus can help you get by with minimal bodily damage. If it helped those little mice in their swimming tests, it may help you make it through the holiday season, your daughter's wedding, or final exams.

BARBERRY

Berberis vulgaris

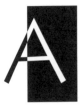s a landscape designer, I've installed thousands of barberry bushes around the United States, but I never used to like them because they're painful to the touch—as the name implies, they're covered with barbs. What I didn't realize and what most homeowners with *berberis* in their front yards still don't know, however, is that the barberry is one of the world's most famous herbal health-givers.

Thirty Plants That Can Save Your Life!

If you have ever done any reading on herbalism, you are bound to have come across the ancient doctrine of signatures. This ancient notion holds that plants which look like an afflicted body part are bound to be good for that part because that is the way God reveals plants' medicinal uses. For example, tomatoes look like a heart and were used to treat heart symptoms.

What does this have to do with our spiny friend? The barberry's wood and roots are a distinctive electric yellow. The first symptom of a bad liver is yellowish skin, and during the days when herbalists followed the doctrine of signatures, liver malfunction was treated with barberry.

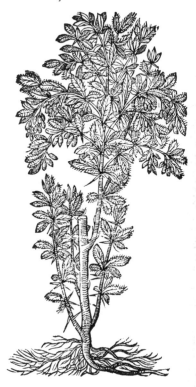

Much to my surprise, the barberry does, in fact, help the liver out in a big way. Its yellow root is used as a hepatic biliary stimulant because some of its elements enhance the flow of bile through the liver and gallbladder. As bile, the detergent of the liver, flows freely, the liver is able to cleanse the blood more effectively and filter out things like artificial preservatives, alcohol, and other environmental toxins. It's one part of the body that you do not want to fool with. When the liver goes, so do you.

But barberry is good for more than the liver. A tidy list of its other uses includes treatment for: alcohol abuse, arthritis, bronchial congestion, cancer, general debility, gallstones, malaria, splenic enlargements, skin diseases, and tumors. It's also effective as a stimulating digestive tonic.

Barberry is no newcomer on the scene of staying well—we are talking about a plant in constant use since before the crucifixion of Christ. Its family is large, with members on every continent, and all over the world barberries are used for maintaining strength and vitality. Modern herbalists feel that barberry root is so powerful that it should only be used occasionally. Like spring cleaning, you only want to do it every once in a while.

In North America, the native barberry is the Oregon grape, *Berberis aquifolium*. It found its way into the pharmacopeia of the United States after physicians learned of it from the Native Americans, and it was brought into common usage when Parke, Davis and Company, of Detroit, Michigan, offered a product containing this plant for sale to physicians in the late 1900s. The Native Americans gathered it in great quantities for tonic purposes. Oregon grape grows naturally with a plant called pipsissewa, and the two plants were used in combination to treat any acute or chronic illness. The Blackfeet Indians peeled the root, dried it, and used it in a tea to stop rectal hemorrhage and dysentery. One recipe for hepatitis included Oregon grape, dandelion, and fennel seed to make the mixture more palatable. The Native Americans also discovered that teas made with Oregon grape root cured people who suffered from recurrent fevers. In a nutshell, they used the Oregon grape to put the whistle back in people who had lost their zip. The point at which we moderns only have enough energy to watch the boob tube is the point at which the medicine man would hand us a bag of Oregon grape root and tell us to start boiling.

BARBERRY. Every once in a while, I give my liver a treat: a healthy dose of barberry. My favorite way to do this is to smear barberry chutney on my morning toast. To make the chutney, add four cups of barberries to two cups of water and cook them down for about ten minutes. After straining the mixture through a spaghetti strainer to get the pits out, cook it down for another ten minutes, combine it with equal parts honey, and keep it in the refrigerator for times when your liver needs special attention.

In the Southwest, Spanish colonials encountered yet another barberry, Palo Amarillo or Fremont's barberry, *Mahonia fremontii*. A close relation to the Oregon grape, it is a tall shrub that looks like a holly tree with blue berries rather than red. Native Americans used it to treat tuberculosis, rheumatism, and jaundice. It was considered a cooling plant, and as such was appropriate for treating any fever, hepatitis and malaria included. In upstate New York, the colonials found a different barberry, the Canadian barberry, *Berberis canadensis*, which they used like all the other barberries around the world. In addition, the berries were cooked into pies and jellies, the tender greens were tossed into salads, and the wood was employed in the making of a bright yellow dye.

The Chinese, who use 17 different barberries in their medicine, have found that there is scientific basis for the plant's reputation in promoting longevity. The principle chemical in barberry is berberine, a snappy item clinically proven to kill bacteria, stop diarrhea and convulsions, stimulate the uterus, and relax the smooth muscles of the intestine. What's more, since berberine is not appreciably absorbed following oral administration, the alkaloids or extracts of plants containing it are often used for the treatment of various intestinal infections, especially bacillary dysentery. It also contains the important anticancer compounds dehydropodophyllotoxin and podophyllotoxin.

Along the lines of prolonging life, many of the barberries have been found to be aphrodisiac in nature—they're apparently so stimulating to the body that all it wants to do is procreate. Epimedium, considered the best in this vein, is said to increase the number of erections that can be had each night, the number of sperm in each ejaculate, and the volume of the ejaculate itself. That's interesting information, since when the body is healthy, a normal sex drive usually results. I guess we would have to call this a side effect—whether it's an unpleasant or a pleasant one is subject to debate.

▼▼▼▼▼▼▼▼▼▼▼▼▼▼▼▼▼▼▼▼▼

BLESSED THISTLE
Cnicus benedictus

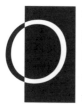

One folk tale of the discovery of blessed thistle's dynamic health-giving and life-saving powers comes to us from the days of Charlemagne. It seems that the emperor was in the middle of one of his pillage-and-plunder routines when his troops were taken ill with a dose of the plague. An angel came to Charlemagne in his sleep and told him that if he were to shoot an arrow into the air, the arrow would land on the plant that would cure his men. The arrow fell on a big old patch of *Cnicus benedictus*, the emperor immediately fed it to the troops, their lives were saved, and the plant was dubbed the blessed thistle.

Herbalists during the days and nights of the knights used blessed thistle to cure not only the plague but also agues and jaundice. The roots soaked in wine created a refreshing cocktail said to knock out bad humors and make the body strong and vital. A blood purifier, it was even eaten as a vegetable when young and tender.

But clearly its greatest fame came from its ability to cure the plague—no small feat. It is mentioned in virtually all the writings issued during times of epidemic infectious diseases, including Shakespeare's *Much Ado About Nothing*. Thomas Brasbridge's 1578 publication *A Poor Man's Jewel* sings the virtues of the blessed thistle and actually goes on to mention angelica as a second-best choice in dealing with the plague. In *Turner's Herbal*, written in 1568, the author recommends the plant as a tonic and stimulant to the whole body as well as one of the best purging agents around.

Along with bloodletting, purging was quite popular in the 16th century. Did you ever wonder why on earth people were purposefully bled? At one time, it was commonly held that sickness was caused by something evil inside the body,

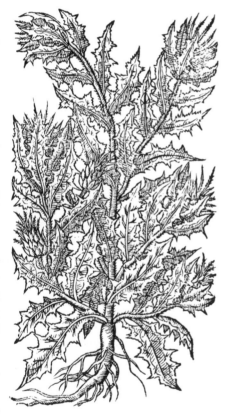

which doctors tried to purge by bleeding their patients or inducing vomiting. Turner was quick to say that blessed thistle emptied out the system with "little pain or discomfort." I don't know about you, but I don't think anything could make spending that kind of time at the porcelain bowl painless other than a big hit of opium. Not to worry, though, you would have to eat a lot of blessed thistle to get the purging effect. In the 19th-century United States, the Shakers, who also used the plant and its roots as a tonic, sweat inducer, and diuretic, found that a double- or triple-strength tea made of blessed thistle would cause a total evacuation of the intestinal tract. Modern research has shown that one of the active ingredients in the plant is indeed a stomach irritant when taken in large quantities. The message here is that a little goes a long way.

Other European herbalists of Turner's day noted the plant's power in strengthening and improving the mind, a feature that should have particular appeal to us today. The pressures of the modern world can strip the mind. This is a fact, and if we take vitamins for the body, why not take something for the mind?

During the Renaissance, blessed thistle was also used to get the milk flowing in nursing mothers, a crucial matter when lack of breast milk meant death to junior. If junior made it to childhood, his mother would use blessed thistle to

Thirty Plants That Can Save Your Life!

worm him before he went to school (it was really bad form to send the kids off to class with a dose of worms). Children and dogs alike got wormed a couple of times a year with blessed thistle.

Culpeper, an herbalist who wrote about blessed thistle in 1652, extolled the same virtues of the plant as did his predecessors. Clearly New Age 400 years before anyone ever thought of playing synthesized space sounds in birthing rooms, Culpeper believed that different plants were ruled by different planets, as were the diseases they cured. Of blessed thistle, he wrote:

By antipathy to other planets, it cures the French pox by antipathy to Venus who governs it. It strengthens the memory and cures deafness by antipathy to Saturn, who hath his fall in Aries which rules the head. It cures quarten agues and other diseases of melancholy, and a dust of choller by sympathy to Saturn.... It also provokes urine, the stopping of which is usually caused by Mars or the moon.

BLESSED THISTLE. *I have to confess that this is one nasty-tasting herb, and a cup of blessed thistle tea is not something I would want to serve the Garden Club. Some herb beverages I can savor, this one I swallow as fast as I can! As my taste buds pitch a fit when they come into contact with it, I make blessed thistle into a syrup to take in the morning. Boil two cups of the herb, fresh or dried, with six cups of water, strain the mixture, and sweeten it with honey. A teaspoon a day keeps the mortician away, or so I like to think.*

Venereal disease, or as Culpeper put it, the "French pox" killed as many Europeans as the plague, and the use of blessed thistle to cure both infectious diseases raises some curious questions which have yet to be answered.

As for blessed thistle's diuretic effects, Gerard agreed in 1597 that the plant "healeth the griping pains of the belly, killeth and expelleth worms, causeth sweat, provoketh urine, and driveth out gravel." What Gerard called "gravel" are gallstones, caused by the improper elimination of waste—the residue collects in the bladder and forms crystals that have to come out eventually.

Taken in small doses, blessed thistle increases urination and sweating, thus flushing the body of toxins contained in it. Doctors of the past century felt diaphoretics, or sweat inducers, cleansed the body of chemical toxins and also bacteria. Physicians found that patients complaining of the early symptoms of a cold or flu could nip it in the bud using blessed thistle. "An infusion made in cold or warm water, if drunk freely, and the patient be kept warm, occasions a plentiful sweat, and promotes the secretions in general," wrote Howard Horton, M.D., in 1879. Horton suggested this method for sparing patients from infectious diseases.

In contemporary herbalism, blessed thistle is still used to treat infectious diseases. It is also used to treat liver and mucous congestion, loss of appetite, dyspepsia, jaundice, and hepatitis. It also lowers fevers, resolves blood clots, and stops bleeding. Its proven ability to speed the body's waste-removing systems, as indicated by increased urination, is what herbalists feel specifically recommends it for us moderns. We take in a lot of trash, which our bodies then have to get rid of. Blessed thistle does the job.

Blessed thistle is readily available at natural food stores and even more readily grown, regardless of where you live. As Thomas Basbridge wrote in 1578, "Blessed thistle expelleth all poyson taken it at the mouth and other corruption that doth hurt and annoye the hart. Therefore I counsel all that have gardens nourish it, that they may have it always to their own use, and the use of their neighbors that lacke it." So plant some! An annual plant, it drops copious quantities of seeds that come up year after year. Order your seeds from a mail-order source and plant them directly in the garden as early as the soil can be worked. The seeds will pop right up, and before you know it, the plants will have reached three feet in height.

The crop should be harvested when the plants break into bloom and either used fresh or hung by the roots to dry in a moisture-free location. When harvesting, pull the plants up by the roots and wash off the dirt. Care should be taken to leave at least five plants in the garden so that they can reseed for next year's crop. As the flower heads on the existing plants dry, you can help the reseeding process by breaking the dry seed heads up and turning them into the soil. This is important to do because birds like the seeds, and if they have a chance at them, your next year's crop will be reduced. Also, the seed comes with "whirlybirds" that catch the wind, and your blessed thistle bed is apt to move around the garden if you don't deal with the seed heads yourself.

BURDOCK

Arctium lappa

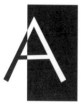

A famous herbalist recently explained to me that the most helpful medicinal herbs are the weeds that insist on living near us! People have been trying to eradicate this "pest" since the first lawn was neatly flattened with a steam roller, and guess who has lost the battle? Despite the onslaught of persnickety lawnkeepers, burdock shows itself every year. If there is truth to the doctrine of signatures that says a plant's appearance indicates its use, then the implication is that eating burdock will make you indestructible. Who knows? The notion is certainly consistent with what the world has to say about burdock.

You may not connect the word *burdock* with the actual plant, but I am certain you have crossed its path before. You may only know it as the weed that refuses to die, but you do know it. It's the plant with the huge, rhubarblike leaves and the tenacious burs that always end up in your kid's or dog's hair. Think of what big hints Mother Nature gave us with this one—it all but carries itself into your house and screams, "Notice me."

Every rose has its thorns, and while the plant may not be pleasing to the lawn fanatic, it is especially pleasing to the body. After doing some research, I think you will agree this is perhaps one of the only plants in the yard that definitely should not be pulled up.

Okay, quiz time. What is a spring tonic and how does it apply to you? In case you drew a blank, here's my answer. Before the advent of grocery stores, trucking, and refrigeration, fresh greens were not available during the winter months. By the time spring rolled around, people were real tired of eating boiled potatoes and dried meats. They looked forward to the first wild greens poking up in the woods and fields, and as soon as these plants stood a few inches over the chilly soil, folks gathered the greens in big pots and boiled them up for "spring tonic."

After eating their first pot of wild weeds, people noticed that they suddenly felt stronger and more energetic; colds that had lingered all winter went away. The water in which the greens had been boiled was always reserved for pregnant women and the ailing, and it came to be known as pot liquor.

The greens are so filled with vitamins and minerals that the water in which they are cooked turns black, and I mean really black. Despite the nasty color and even nastier taste, people eagerly drank the pot liquor because it made them feel better, and being in good shape to plant the year's crops was a life-or-death issue.

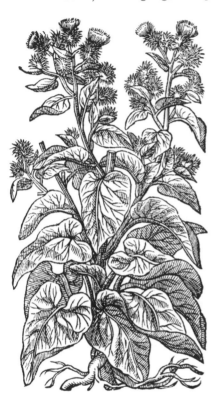

This business of gathering the first greens of spring for health is as old as the hills and an American tradition. In time, people became adept at telling which greens available at the first blast of spring were good for what: dandelions for the liver, plantain for the stomach, and burdock root for overall strength and vitality.

The long, thin taproot of the burdock plant, the anchor that keeps it so firmly attached to the earth, was the part used by our ancestors for spring tonic. Gerard, our 17th-century herbalist friend, noted that burdock made a first-class root vegetable with the added benefit of stirring up a little lust. This notion is also held by the Chinese, and their research has concluded that it does indeed raise the libido. Remember, healthy people have healthy sex drives. What's more, the root can be as much as 45 percent inulin, a sugar of great interest to diabetics.

The Pennsylvania Dutch, who have made a lifestyle of preserving the old-time culture, still gather greens for spring tonic, and burdock root is always included. They also use the one-year-old roots of burdock, or *gladda wartzel* as they call it, in tea which they take both internally as a general blood purifier and externally as a wash for dandruff. They ingest the seeds for kidney ailments and make a tea of them for use as an external wash for skin problems, including first-aid for cuts and burns.

Burdock seems to be a plant that when taken a little at a time, in increasing amounts, cleanses the body of toxins through its mildly laxative and diuretic effects. Whose job is toxic-waste clean-up? The liver. Bad skin was traditionally believed to be a sign of a poorly functioning liver, and so when burdock was used internally for skin problems, it was really more to treat the liver, the source of the problem.

Burdock's considerable reputation as a blood purifier is also related to its function in stimulating the liver and kidneys, because these are the organs which tidy up the blood. This same cleansing property accounts for its widespread use in the treatment of snakebite, which seems to have been much more of an issue years back when people spent most of their time out in the fields.

The Chinese, who, like many people around the world, believe that burdock is good for the lungs, find it most effective in treating pneumonia, sore throats, and chronic coughs. Their scientists, by the by, have shown that burdock has anti-tumor and anti-cancer activities, a finding which dovetails with their use of the plant in treating cancers. It has also been proven to have an antimicrobial effect due to the polyacetylenes it contains. The Chinese have found burdock extracts to be antifungal and antibacterial as well, making it the perfect remedy for a lung infection.

BURDOCK. I've adopted a tasty Japanese recipe for burdock salad. Peel the brown outer skin off the root. The Japanese would then cut the root into toothpick shapes, but I'm too lazy for that, so I zap it in the food processor into slices the thickness of dimes. In a separate bowl, mix four teaspoons of soy sauce, two teaspoons of sesame oil, one teaspoon of rice vinegar, one teaspoon of sliced spring onion, one teaspoon of sesame seeds, and two tablespoons of honey. Pour the dressing over the sliced burdock, stick it in the fridge, and eat it for as long as it lasts. The more it marinates, the better it tastes.

In days before inoculation and antibiotics, measles was a dangerous and often fatal disease, and an epidemic could devastate an entire community. In a 1962 volume of a West Virginia folklore society's journal, an informant born in Wetzel County at the turn of the century offered a choice measles treatment. According to this man, one Frank King, "Measles may sometimes be dangerous if they tend to go inside instead of breaking out on the surface as they should. Sheep nanny tea (made from sheep manure) can be used to make the measles break out as can a brew made by boiling burdock roots in sweetened water."

The same guidance can be found in a number of books on Southern folk medicine. In parts of Georgia, the roots were soaked in whiskey, and the cocktail was taken either to get rid of measles or to avoid getting them in the first place. I'll take burdock tea over sheep poop cappuccino any day.

The Chinese go along with the Southerners' notion and go one step further, stating that burdock, or *niu bang zi*, is good not only for measles but also for all other infectious diseases, especially those that appear in epidemic fashion. On the proof side of things, they have shown that burdock tea has a serious inhibitory effect on a number of obnoxious bacteria and fungi.

Most of us moderns work in group situations where when one person gets a cold, everybody gets it. "It's going around the office" has replaced "a bad humor is sweeping the village," and burdock should be brought back as a shield against the diseases air conditioners spit in our faces while we're sitting in our cubicles. A healthy addition to any teapot, the plant is an overall strengthener, a tonic that makes the body robust. And that's what it's all about, getting the body strong so that you can do what you want to do.

Obtaining burdock is not an issue—it can be found at any herb seller's and in just about any abandoned lot. The problem is getting the thing out of the ground. To accomplish this, wait until your area has had several rainy days so that the ground is good and wet. With a deep spade, start digging a foot away from the plant. Keep working until you feel the plant pull away from the soil, then give it a good yank. The whole plant can be used in the tonic, fresh or dried, although fresh is, of course, better. It stays green year-round, so getting it fresh won't be an issue, but because burdock is most packed with healing in the late fall, it is best to gather burdock then.

Burdock may not be appreciated in the lawn, but it is certainly a healthful plant. Why fight it? If you are looking for a ground cover that won't quit, consider using this fuzzy and fantastic plant. All you need to do is go for a walk in the woods, and when you get home, pull the burs off your clothes, and toss them in some garden soil.

CINNAMON

Cinnamomum zeylanicum

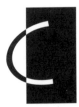innamon was one of the first trade spices of the ancient world. Biblical references indicate that merchants carried the Asian spice all the way from Ceylon to Palestine—that's a 24-hour airplane trip today—before the pyramids were built. The English word *cinnamon* derives from the Hebrew word *kinnamon*, and the spice is mentioned in Psalms, Proverbs, Ezekiel, and Revelations. Moses, the patriarch of patriarchs,

Thirty Plants That Can Save Your Life!

commanded the children of Israel to anoint the tabernacle, the vessels of the tabernacle, and the priests themselves with ointments made of cinnamon. Let's remember that the stuff was hauled from beyond India without the help of jet engines, and the Phoenicians and Arabians who hauled it weren't working for peanuts. Why did Moses specify cinnamon and others pay the price it cost? Because it was and still is special. There is something about cinnamon that made it worth any expense.

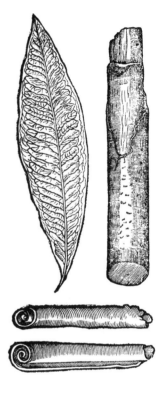

Moses was not cinnamon's first admirer, and many others were to follow, agreeing that it was the superlative body splash and more. The ancients Theophrastus, Herodotus, Galen, Dioscorides, Pliny, and Strabo all mention it. Cinnamon ranked in value with gold, ivory, and frankincense, and was among the most costly offerings in the temple of Apollo in Miletus in 243 B.C. The early Egyptians used cinnamon in their embalming mixtures, and Chinese medicinal use of the spice dates back 4,700 years.

The Arabians discovered that when you boil out the oils contained in a plant, those oils purvey the scent of said plant, be it roses or cinnamon, and so they imported cinnamon from the Orient, distilled the fragrant oil out, and sold the more easily transported substance to the Europeans. In this form, the spice made its way from Arabia to Venice, and from Venice to all points in Europe. If cinnamon sticks were special, cinnamon oil was considered bonus deluxe.

Cinnamon is the bark and twigs of a number of related plants that have one thing in common: cinnamon oil. The plants rarely reach higher than 30 feet; the leaves are deep green and the blossoms usually white. Once the trees are six or seven years old, the bark is peeled off into so-called cinnamon sticks. Ground into powder, they yield what we find in cans on the grocer's shelf. Aside from a great-tasting dusting for doughnuts, we don't see cinnamon as being very special anymore. This is unfortunate.

Cinnamon is one of the oldest tonic plants on the globe. The world may not agree politically, but in the realm of tonics, all acknowledge that cinnamon is good for health. The Chinese feel that cinnamon used on a daily basis over a long period of time will improve the complexion, giving the taker a more robust, stronger, and more youthful appearance. One Chinese ancient said that if you took cinnamon with toads' brains for seven years, you would be able to walk on water, look young forever, and never die. While you may have a problem getting your hands on a pound of toads' brains, the active ingredient, cinnamon, is readily available.

Where there's smoke, there's fire, and behind most folk tales, there's some measure of truth. The daily use of cinnamon could well improve your health. The Chinese believe that cinnamon heats up a cold body, improves the circulation, and generally gets the blood rushing around, stoking up the waning fire, if you will, and they prescribe it for loss of vigor, whether due to stress, aging, or illness. They believe the spice warms the kidneys and cures impotence, weak legs, and backache. Specifically, cinnamon is held supreme for blood deficiencies that leave one feeling weak.

CINNAMON. Nothing beats cinnamon tea when I'm feeling sluggish or run down. Take four cinnamon sticks, or two teaspoons of cinnamon, and add to two cups of boiling water. Let it boil for ten minutes, then sweeten to taste. While the tea is boiling, I like to change into something comfortable, place several trashy, celebrity-bashing magazines on the sofa with a blanket, and turn off the phone. I take my tea to the sofa and sit down for a good read. After my second cup, I settle down for a nap, and I always wake up ready to go.

In India, cinnamon is used to flavor sweet treats, but every villager also knows that chewing on the cinnamon stick is a powerful treatment for the monthlies. The spice, which stimulates the uterine muscles, is also used in difficult deliveries due to inadequate contractions. A painkiller as well as a uterine stimulant, cinnamon is essentially the herbal equivalent of many over-the-counter menstrual medications. The Chinese, who along with other Asians use it as a treatment for PMS, agree that cinnamon promotes regular and easy menstruation.

Did you ever notice that after eating a cinnamon-powdered doughnut you couldn't help but love the whole world? And you thought it was your blood sugar reaching an acceptable level! Cinnamon has been used as a tranquilizer since before Western civilization became civilized (that is to say if it ever did).

The source of this sedative effect is the cinnamaldehyde contained in cinnamon powder and, more powerfully, in cinnamon oil, which has been proven to tranquilize both animals and human beings. In some interesting Chinese research, scientists discovered that they were able to neutralize the effects of phenobarbital and methamphetamine in mice with a matching dose of cinnamaldehyde. The same chemical was found to relieve pain in mice. Since overcharged nerves do present a threat to life and, as they say, stress kills, a hot cup of relaxing cinnamon tea may be just what the herbalist ordered.

The folk treatment for bronchial asthma in various parts of Asia, this same cinnamon tea has been found by researchers to stop most sufferers' attacks. More and more, asthma is being linked to emotional upset, and the calming nature of the substance may be at the root of this cure.

In days gone by and even today, a high fever can be the end of you—if nothing else, elevated body temperature can make you feel out of whack. One of the Chinese treatments for fever is a dose of cinnamon, and indeed, research has shown that after being injected with salmonella and typhoid, mice, the poor creatures, had a reduction in temperature when treated with cinnamaldehyde. This may be due to cinnamon's ability to open up the blood vessels. Scientific validation aside, the news to you is that if you have a fever, cinnamon is likely to reduce it.

The world we live in is filled with disease. Let's face it, everywhere you look you see people sneezing and coughing, and usually on you. When you only get two weeks off a year, who wants to spend that precious time in bed watching reruns? The main folk use of cinnamon has been fighting infection, and following the custom of taking it after exposure to an illness in the aim of not getting sick yourself might not be a bad idea.

Here are some facts, not theories, facts. Cinnamon oil has exhibited antifungal, antiviral, bactericidal, and larvicidal activities. Specifically, ingredients in cinnamon kill escherichia coli, staphylococcus aureus, salmonella, the Asian flu virus A, and echo virus. What does this mean? These are all nasty bacteria that can make you exceptionally ill. Salmonella causes food poisoning, escherichia coli causes Montezuma's revenge, and staphylococcus aureus causes lesions, pustules, and boils that can be terminal if they spread to the organs. Not a pretty picture, but the good news is that cinnamon has been proven to suppress their growth, and the growth of several other gram-positive bacteria.

Not surprisingly, the folk belief that cinnamon can stop bacteria, fungus, and viruses from attacking food or persons is absolutely true. From now on, whenever you come in contact with snot-nosed children harboring all of the above, have yourself a cup of hot cinnamon tea.

Could there be more from this all-in-one-pharmacy plant? Yes. "For pe stomak. Dis driep vp pe ille humoure of pe stomak, and hit comfortep it and strength it." A Middle English translation of a famous Latin herbal called *Macer Floridus de viribus herbarum*, written somewhere around the ninth century, asserts in its easy-to-read style that cinnamon gets rid of bad things that hang out in the stomach, calms it down, and makes it stronger. As a stomach remedy, cinnamon hails supreme, and Macer's claim is actually quite in keeping with the research done of late. If your stomach is upset by a bug of sorts, cinnamon will kill it (the bug). If your stomach is all in a knot, cinnamon will relax it. People in the ninth century knew more about cinnamon than we do! And we think of ourselves as so worldly.

You know where to get cinnamon. The plant isn't grown much in the United States, although several locales would suit it fine. A hot-weather plant, it would have to be grown in a greenhouse or in the sunnier parts of the country. Though the plant isn't especially appropriate for the garden, ground cinnamon and cinnamon sticks are easy to find in any grocery or health food store. An herbal hint—the best cinnamon comes from the Chinese pharmacist. The extra-good news is that unlike many of our tonic plants, this one actually tastes nice and adds a pleasant flavor to a homemade cure-all.

▼▼▼▼▼▼▼▼▼▼▼▼▼▼▼▼▼▼▼▼▼▼▼▼

DANDELION
Taraxacum officinale

ven people who only see greenery in public parks know dandelions. The plant, which is native to Asia, has made the entire planet its home. Most of us consider it a curse, but we shouldn't. The dandelion is a leader in the tonic hall of fame.

As is obvious from its global colonization, the plant is both tough and adaptable. It grows in a funnel shape so that any falling water rolls right down to the plant's center, towards the root, where it is needed. The dandelion's parachutelike seeds blown from the plant in every direction are another adaptation that makes it impossible to eradicate. One white seed head hit with a gust of wind can start 200 or more new plants. It's built to last, I like to say.

Like other top tonic plants the world has known, the dandelion is surrounded by legends. The plant has been said to predict just about anything you can imagine, from the weather to the number of children a bride will have. Many people use the existence of these superstitious beliefs as a reason to discredit a plant's use in folk medicine, but this is a mistake. When a culture bothers to create myths around a plant, it is because the plant has some proven power. Let's take a trip around the world to see what people know about the dandelion.

The dandelion came to the region we now call New Mexico with the Spaniards, and chicoria, as it was known in the 1820s, was used for both food and medicine. To cure heart trouble, the blooms were collected and boiled in water until the water turned bright yellow. The liquid was then allowed to sit out of doors overnight, and a glassful was drunk every morning for a solid month.

Travel a few miles over to San Ildefonso Pueblo, and we find village mothers grinding dandelion leaves, applying the paste to broken bones, and wrapping wounds with bandages encrusted with fresh leaves to speed healing. In Santa Clara, ground dandelion leaves traditionally were added to dough and applied to bad bruises to take the blood out.

Moving northward on the map and backwards in the history books, our next stop is French Canada. In 1748, the Swede, Peter Kalm, traveled by foot and canoe across the wilderness from the outermost British fort, Fort Nicholson in Albany, to the closest French fort, Fort St. Frederic. Our friend Peter was a botanist, at least at heart, and guess what he found in French Canada? The dandelion. He said that the Frenchmen had carried the plant to the New World and were using its bitter roots in a healthful tonic salad.

Let's go downward on the map and time line to Pennsylvania, mid-18th century. Here we find a large group of Mennonites who had fled religious persecution in Germany and brought *pissabet* or *bittera tzelaut*, the dandelion, with them. When they ate the young plant as an early spring tonic, they were being smart, as the leaf contains six or seven times more units of vitamin A per ounce than lettuce or carrots. It's also a source of vitamins B and C. In addition, the Mennonites used dandelion roots as the chief home remedy for kidney or liver trouble as manifested by jaundice or yellowing of the skin.

Next stop, a mid-19th-century Shaker village. A very interesting sect which came from England and picked up some converts along the way, the Shakers were into helping people, doing community service, and generally making the world a nicer place. When they got involved in the herb business, they became

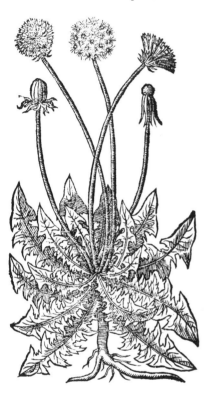

famous for their health products. The Shakers felt that dandelion roots helped the liver, and from the records of their sales of dandelion products, the public, who commissioned them to make the stuff, agreed. These communities of do-gooders didn't believe in having sex, and with the universal hobby taken out of the picture, they had a lot of time to get real clear on which plant was good for what condition. Their recommendation is a serious one.

Last North American stop, the Delaware Valley where seeds from the white man's plants spread to Native Americans' backyards. The Delaware Indians quickly got into the act and deemed the dandelion a most excellent spring tonic. The Tewa tribe found the same to be true and prized the leaves for spring salads.

As in New Mexico, the dandelion arrived in South America with the Spaniards. In Costa Rica, which is famous for its herb markets, dandelions are sold for treating diabetes. In Guatemala, we find not one but two different dandelions sold by the fresh medicine man: a narrow-leaved dandelion, called *diente de leon*, as a tonic for all-over body health, and a second variety, called *amargon*, as a salad green and blood strengthener, especially in the case of anemia. In Brazil, the Portuguese brother of this Guatemalan herbsman says the same thing—dandelion is a blood purifier, with the added benefits of treating liver problems, scurvy, and any urinary complaint that might be present.

Not surprisingly, the dandelion has been used in European and Asian folk medicine for hundreds of years. The Chinese have been working with it longer than anyone else, and their scientific research has proven that the annoying weed has diuretic, hypoglycemic, antispasmodic, anticancer, antibacterial, and antifungal effects on the body. The dandelion is mentioned in all sorts of ancient documents, including the *Pentsao* and the Tang *Materia Medica*, as both food and medicine, and the Chinese have been using it to treat breast cancer for more than 1,100 years. They also use it for: abscesses, appendicitis, boils, caries, dermatitis, fever, inflammation, leucorrhea, liver ailments, mastitis, scrofula, snakebites, and stomachaches.

Chinese scientists have discovered that dandelion extracts have an in vitro bactericidal effect against a number of really nasty bacteria, including those responsible for diphtheria, tuberculosis, and pneumonia. Not to mention the fact that they control that ever-so-deadly staphylococcus aureus (staph infection) when it has invaded the body. The Chinese also found that the plant's roots, leaves, juice, and extracts are effective in treating other infections, including chronic bronchitis and hepatitis, with few side effects.

It stands to reason that if the liver is in good functioning order, cleaning out all the toxins known to cause cancer, dandelion may indeed be a cancer preventative herb. As far as staying well in general goes, the plant has been proven to kill bacteria, in effect purifying the blood, which is what people around the world have been saying for centuries.

Dandelions are not plants that you have to mail-order or buy at the garden center—all you could ever use are available free for the picking. Most of your neighbors will be more than happy to share their bounty of the not-so-ornamental blooms, but remember the companies that spray lawns are not your friends when it comes to collecting dandelions. The stuff they put down is toxic to all involved, and using dandelions treated with their spray of death could lead to yours. Only collect dandelions from insecticide- and herbicide-free ground. You can also buy them at the natural food store, but by the time you have driven there, parked the car, shopped, and made the return trip, you could have picked some fresh herb. For our tonic, dandelions are best collected in the fall after they

DANDELION. It works best for me to fit my use of herbs into my pre-existing routine. Good or bad, for 15 years I have had coffee every morning, and in recent years I've modified my routine by adding a little dandelion. Gather a salad bowl of dandelion plants—roots, leaves, and all—wash them, and put them in the oven. Set the oven at 250° and leave them in until they are brown and crispy, about 30 minutes. Grind the whole kit and caboodle into a powder in a food processor. In a zip-lock bag, mix one cup of this dandelion powder with one cup of ground coffee, and use the mixture to make the morning brew.

have spent the season soaking up sunshine, or power, as I like to think about it. Ideally, the whole plant should be gathered and tossed into your tonic pot nice and fresh, but it can also be dried in the sun for later use.

I grow a patch of dandelions to have on hand whenever I need them, and if you like those chic bitter greens offered at expensive restaurants, dandelions are the easiest ones to grow. Go gather some roots and plant a good row in the garden. Once they are well established, which won't take long, cover the plants with straw for two weeks before harvesting the leaves. The absence of light blanches the leaves a whitish yellow and reduces the bitter contents so that the plant is more pleasant to eat.

▼▼▼▼▼▼▼▼▼▼▼▼▼▼▼▼▼▼▼▼▼▼

DATE

Phoenix dactylifera

he date is mentioned in the Bible no fewer than 42 times, an amazing number to befit an amazing plant. You may have thought that it was just another ingredient in Christmas puddings and cakes, but this simplistic view has got to go.

The plant and its fruit had their start in ancient Mesopotamia, the cradle of civilization. A coin issued in Palestine from the year 175 B.C. bears a date palm tree on one side, and so prized has the fruit been throughout Jewish history that the Hebrew word for date, *tamar* or *tamarah*, is still used as a name for female children. The date palm grew in such abundance in what we now call modern Israel that the area from the Sea of Galilee to the Dead Sea was one huge date forest.

As with many highly medicinal plants, the date palm figures prominently in the mythology of a number of cultures. The ancient Greeks dedicated it to the god Apollo. Jews believe that it was the tree of knowledge in the Garden of Eden; Moslems believe that it was created by Mohammed. In Christianity, the date palm became a symbol of martyrdom, and the souls of Christian martyrs were said to be carried to heaven on palm fronds. All cultures agree: dates are a magical food.

Date palm trees start bearing fruit at six or seven years, though they don't reach maturity until their thirtieth year. Once fully mature, a date palm will continue to produce for two centuries. Like holly trees, date palm trees come in both male and female, and a good-sized female is capable of producing hundreds of pounds of dates. The date is both a cultivated plant and one that grows wild from India through Western Asia, the Middle East, and all of Northern Africa.

At times in the Near East, this, the earliest known palm, has been quite literally the staff of life. An Arabic saying holds that there are as many uses for the date palm as there are days in the year. According to Herodotus, the ancient Arabians used it to make bread, wine, and honey, and people could quite literally survive on nothing but the date tree. During times of war, the worst thing that an enemy could do to a tribe was destroy the male palm trees, thus ruining the possibility of fruit. In fact, so important was the date palm to early Near Eastern

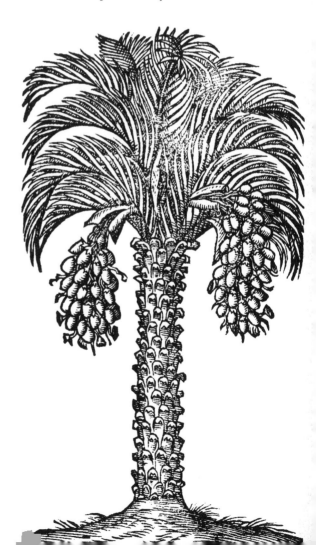

societies that it made its way into the ornamentation of their most prominent buildings, and from the time of the construction of Solomon's Temple forward, columns mimicked the date palm's elegant terminal buds.

In Saudi Arabia, the stones of the fruit are still ground and roasted for date coffee, which is said to be a good substitute for the ordinary kind. Distilling the fruits yields a spirit called *lagbi* or *rajura-no-darn*. Moreover, the kernel of the date can be ground up or soaked in water for several days and fed to camels, cows, and goats. This date pit meal is said to be so nutritious that it does the animals more good than their usual fare of wheat and barley. These same seeds can be turned into stylish accessories for an evening on the town—livestock feed and fashion statement all in one!

Throughout the Middle East, male date palms are tapped much the way Americans tap maple trees to make syrup, and a single tree will yield three or four quarts of sap a day for several weeks. The sweet juice that exudes from the palms can be drunk for refreshment as is or fermented into a highly intoxicating beverage. Left to ferment even further, this spirit then forms what is known as *arrak*.

Strabo, Herodotus, and Pliny all credit the ancient Babylonians with thinking up this cocktail. Biblical mentions of an alcoholic beverage stronger than wine could very well refer to male date palm hooch, which is said to be very diuretic and cleansing to the body.

Beyond the fact that every part of the tree finds its way into some sort of food, be it for man or beast, the fruit itself has been recognized as a powerful health giver. True, it's high in sugar, but the people who live with the tree and its fruit have observed that there is something more to the date than a quick sugar fix. The date contains some substance with the power to restore health to those who are failing. The Arabs, who are still in intimate contact with the fruit, believe that it somehow traps the power of the sun and that this trapped power is capable of healing. Traditional Arabic medicine uses the date to relieve coughs, to clean out the system, to regulate urination, and to enhance fertility. Green dates are reputed to be both aphrodisiac and tonic, date kernels are made into a poultice to treat genital ulcers, and the juice of boiled dates is given to invalids to restore their overall strength and vigor.

DATE. I find that having a steady supply of dates in the house assures a constant intake on my part. I am essentially a reformed sugar junkie—I've merely cleaned up my sugar source! Dates can be used instead of sugar in almost any recipe. Grind the dates in the handy food processor, and use the paste one for one as a sugar substitute. Do this, and when you sit down for a slice of cake, you'll be doing yourself some service. My favorite treat in this life is made by substituting dates for the carrots in recipes for carrot cake.

Maimonides, physician to a sultan who lived in the twelfth century, was very fond of prescribing the date for health. It seems that the sultan had several hundred wives and believed in visiting them all as often as his royal schedule would allow. Bedding 200 wives was, of course, a taxing proposition, and the doctor's recommendation for keeping all parts in working order always started with dates as a base. Maimonides felt that dates gave force and vitality to those who ate them. He should know, his number-one patient had a complicated social agenda!

The date appeared in Europe sometime before the life of Christ, among the cargo of ambitious Arab traders. Although the Greeks and Romans enjoyed the fruit in orgiastic pastry parties, people in the know also used it to preserve their health. According to Gerard, dates were "good for those that spit blood, for such as have bad stomachs, and for those also that be troubled with the bloody flux." He also recommended them for sore throats, weak lungs, feeble spleens, failing livers, and flagging libidos. What's more, he wrote: "The ashes of the date stones have a binding quality, they heal puffies in the eyes, Staphylomata, and falling away for the haire of the eye lids." I don't know about you, but I really worry about losing my eyelid hairs, and after spending two decades sweating it out, I will at last be able to get a good night's sleep, thanks to Gerard.

At the risk of offending, which doesn't bother me that much, I will point out that Gerard, like Maimonides, felt that dates procured "lust of the body." This is important because people who have strong bodies have healthy sex desires, and people who don't, don't. The modern phenomena of being so stressed out that even the thought of doing the deed doesn't occur is more and more common. Our rough-and-tumble lives take so much out of the human body and mind that the sex desire goes right out the window. Dates will bring it back.

The ancients and not-so ancients were all in agreement on one thing: dates enhance vigor. The day-to-day grind strips this from us, and as our doctor friends said in the *Yellow Emperor's Inner Classic*, we need more than prayers to stay vital.

Throughout history, people have eaten dates for strength. How did we lose track of what was once common knowledge? That's another book, but for the purpose of this one, which is making a tonic to keep us fit as a fiddle, we will take note of dates. They, of course, are available at every grocery store, and unbeknownst to some, their pits will easily sprout and produce date palm trees. The palm is quite hardy, and if you live south of North Carolina, and have both a male and a female tree, yours will probably bear fruit. However, they are not extensively grown outside of California, which is a pity, because in terms of a dooryard fruit tree, none could be easier or more productive. Remember, one bearing-age female can produce several hundred pounds of fruit, which is more than enough for you and yours.

ECHINACEA

Echinacea purpurea

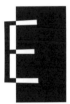chinacea, our next ingredient, is relatively new to most of the world. An indigenous North American plant used first by the Native Americans and then by the pioneers, echinacea is today most commonly found in flower gardens. As a landscape designer, I planted thousands of these plants without knowing the incredible story behind their use and even more astounding reputation. Take a good look and see if you don't have some in your flower garden.

When the first colonists arrived in North America, they were confronted with a multitude of unpleasant things: diseases, insects, and big snakes, to mention a few. The snakes were a special problem as walking around in their territory was part of the plan. Early on the colonials were on the lookout for indigenous plants that could help them survive a snakebite. Those they had known in Europe were far, far away, and the colonists had to make do with what was available. Among the medicinal plants they discovered in use by the Native Americans was echinacea. Different varieties were used by different tribes according to their locations, but they all had one thing in common: they were effective in combating the viper's sting. Somehow, echinacea sped up the process of pumping poison out of the body through the liver and kidneys. Indeed, most life-threatening illnesses were treated with these "snake roots," and in time their powers were thought to be nothing short of miraculous.

As the colonists moved westward, they came into contact with other Native Americans and the plants they used for doctoring. From this exchange of information, new plants were "discovered" and eventually accepted into the stuffed-shirt medical communities safely tucked away on the East Coast and in Europe.

Here's an illustration of how that exchange went down. A certain H. C. F. Meyer, a German country doctor, became aware of echinacea and began using it as the main ingredient in a commercial concoction he called Meyer's Blood Purifier. So convinced was Meyer of echinacea's power to save that he tried to take the information to the medical establishment back east. His intentions were good, but his presentation needed a little work. He offered to let a snake bite him at a medical conference (he would provide the snake or the doctors could collect their own), and he would then cure himself with nothing but echinacea.

You can imagine the pompous physicians sitting at their professional gathering, pressed collars on one and all, with some dust-trail healer screaming outside their window, "Hey, I'll let this here snake bite me, and this here plant will make me right as rain." Well, needless to say, the doctors shut the window and went back to their meeting. Their loss.

Meyer made his offer again, this time to two doctors named King and Lloyd, eclectics who belonged to an herbal branch of medicine now extinct. In a classic example of listening to the message and not the messenger, these two doctors took Dr. Meyer's advice and looked into echinacea's power. Despite initial doubts about the new plant's abilities, it was introduced into the *Materia Medica* in 1887 and enjoyed quite a reputation in the heyday of herb-based medicines.

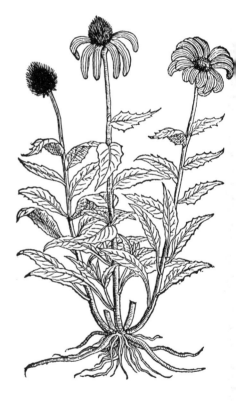

Native to the plains of the United States, echinacea grows wild nowhere else in the world, except for a few sparse patches in southern Canada. It made its way to Europe in the 17th century and was given the name echinacea from the Greek *echinos* (sea urchin or hedgehog) in reference to its spiny flower. Although the plant has caught on and is now one of the most popular herbal remedies in Europe, its history is in North America, and most of the folkloric information about it comes from Native Americans.

The Plains Indians used echinacea to treat toothaches, sore throats, coughs, and infections. Their preferred method was to suck on the root. Did you ever notice the lymph nodes under your chin and how when you get sick they swell up? Well, your lymph glands are located there so that they can pump out immunity cells to mix along with whatever else passes between your lips. They're the first defense in knocking out illness and eliminating toxins as they enter the mouth. Some researchers now feel that chewing on echinacea root is the best way to use the immunity booster as echinacea actually activates the saliva and disease-fighting resources in the mouth so that they can attack anything coming in. The old custom may be the best custom.

The Sioux Indians applied the freshly scraped root of the black sampson or purple coneflower, *Echinacea angustifolia*, as a poultice against hydrophobia caused by the bites of rabid animals. The Cheyenne used the plant for sore mouths, the Choctaws for coughs, the Comanche for sore throats, the Crow for colds, the Kiowas for both sore throats and colds, and the Delaware for venereal diseases. The common denominator here is that the plant was used to treat infection, and science has borne this one out.

Echinacea is the most researched plant in the modern herbal world. It may have taken Dr. Meyer's making an arse of himself, but eventually people took the cotton out of their ears. Here is what echinacea has been found to do: it stimulates the production of leukocytes, the white blood cells that fight infection in the body, and assists the phagocytes in doing their job, which is engulfing toxins, packaging them off, and preparing them for disposal. These cellular M.P.s also remove damaged cells and any other irregularities. Essentially they are trash collectors and quality controllers. If a cell isn't looking right, they zap it. If there is some waste in the corner, they collect it and put it down the shoot.

ECHINACEA. This is a tea plant, and I prefer the fresh herb to the dried hands down. Take two teaspoons of the loose leaves and drop them into two cups of boiling water. Turn the heat off and allow the mixture to infuse for a bit. Drink it when it has cooled down enough. Another use for the leaves, when still tender, is to add them to any salad. With a pair of scissors, cut them into thin strips to scatter over the rest of the greens. The leaves are tender in the spring—the rest of the year is tea time.

Echinacea, which has a mild antibiotic effect, helps protect cells during infection and prevents pathogens, bacteria, and viruses from entering in the first place. The plant both stimulates the properdin/complement system, which likewise helps the body control and prevent infections, and increases production of alpha-1 and alpha-2 gamma globulins, which prevent viral and other infections as does echinacea's interferonlike action.

The message is that echinacea does, in fact, do what the Indians said it did. We moderns don't have to deal with the toxic venom of the snake, but we do have to deal with the toxic venom of contemporary living, and studies indicate that echinacea is just as effective in the latter realm as it was in the former.

Thirty Plants That Can Save Your Life!

You can buy echinacea from any herb seller, but this is a grand waste of money. For the price of one ounce, you can get an entire plant and have echinacea for free right outside your door. The plant is a perennial, and once you plant it, it spreads all over the place. This one is easy to grow. After you've gotten your hands on the plant, the time to harvest is fall.

Echinacea root is used most frequently in modern herbalism, and in order to collect it, you have to destroy the plant. The stems and leaves are just as medicinal, and some feel that they are, in fact, a bit safer for daily use than the oh-so-powerful root. One herbalist, Eric Pollard, told me that the root is such a strong medicine that it should only be used when one finds oneself sick, which isn't going to happen to us anymore once we have our tonic! So you don't have to destroy your plants in the fall—clip them down, and use the stems and leaves in your tonic pot.

▼▼▼▼▼▼▼▼▼▼▼▼▼▼▼▼▼▼▼▼▼▼▼

FIG
Ficus carica

he fig is the original world traveler. A native of Asia Minor, it is now cultivated in temperate countries everywhere on earth. Not only do people like to eat it, but they have also found that it makes the whole body stronger.

Despite the well-known story that Adam and Eve covered their secret parts with leaves torn from the tree, the leaves exude a copious and extremely irritating sap which can even cause blistering, and it's unlikely that the troubled pair donned fig tree outfits more than once. The fruit, on the other hand, are used as treatments for a variety of specific ailments and as restoratives of energy and vitality.

Not only is the fig the first plant cited by name in the Bible, it also gets cited 57 times after that. The fruit grew extensively in the Middle East in biblical times, as it does now, and the custom of planting a fig tree in the corner of the orchard as mentioned in Luke is still practiced in the sandy lands today. The use of figs for healing predates the Bible; it receives several mentions in that famous book. Hezekial, an Israelite king, was said to have been cured of a cancerous

Fig

47

growth with the fruit of a fig. Science has shown that the king's cure may be more than a tale! We will talk about the fruit's use in cancer therapy later, but make a note that in the modern arena figs have been proven to be an effective treatment for cancer.

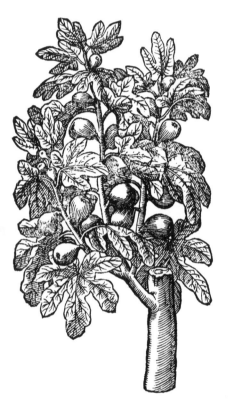

In the Bible, the Children of Israel are continually threatened and rewarded with mentions of the fig. If they act nice, their figs will do well, and if they act badly, their fig trees will die. This shows how important the fig tree was to people. God didn't threaten them with dead petunias. He went for the gusto, for the plant that kept them alive.

The Arabs have used figs for food and medicine for thousands of years. The ancient king Mithrydates in 1551 B.C. proclaimed figs a health tonic, and their repeated mentions in the *Arabian Nights* hint at the pleasure derived from the plant. Traditional Arabian medicine uses figs, which the Arabs believe to be diuretic, laxative, and emollient, to treat conjunctivitis, leprosy, and hemorrhoids. An anise-flavored liquor of the fermented fruits is said to be an excellent tonic.

Most notably, the Arabs see the fig as incredibly strengthening to the body, building stamina and vigor. They also believe that eating figs will make you have lots of children, so if big families are not it for you, better take precautions.

The fig was an instant hit when imported to Rome, and by the year A.D. 23, the Roman naturalist Pliny was writing about its health-giving properties. The life of a gladiator was one where winning was a priority and losing meant death. Under the circumstances, the professional athletes of the day took every element of their personal fitness regime rather seriously. Pliny noted that these ancient sports warriors were fed a diet of figs to bring on incredible strength and stamina. Hey, if they were good enough for the gladiators, they're good enough for me!

During the days of the Roman Empire, 29 B.C. through A.D. 395, figs were

Thirty Plants That Can Save Your Life!

given to and carried by guests at social functions. It seems that the women wore necklaces made of figs—the edible panties of the era—and the men carried phallic sculptures carved from fig wood. This should tell you something about what the Romans thought of the fig. It filled you with vitality in all areas, including the bedroom.

Today we see food and medicine as two separate items, but in days gone by, they were one and the same. I was talking to an African American herbalist recently, and she made an excellent point that we don't seem to remember: you are what you eat. If you eat powerful foods like the fig, you become powerful. If you eat dead foods like chips and french onion dip, you become dead. Pretty simple if you ask me.

Our friend Gerard would probably agree. He recommended figs for ailments of the throat and lungs, for tumors and skin problems from freckles and warts to smallpox and leprosy, for hemorrhoids and kidney stones, and for toothaches, among other maladies. But I think Gerard summed it all up when he said that figs preserve us from all pestilence. This is old English for figs keep us in tip-top condition.

Getting back to my favorite topic, bathroom talk, Gerard along with the rest of the world also felt that figs clean you out. If you have ever eaten one too many figs, you know what he meant. But this cleaning out process is a wonderful—note, I didn't say pleasant—thing. When we get all the garbage out of our system, our immunity functions don't have to work so hard and can focus on killing the little buggers that enter our bodies and cause problems. Actually, the fig's much-touted power to improve overall health and vigor may be due to its ability to promote regularity, which, though no one likes to point this out, is very important.

FIG. My favorite way to consume this heavenly fruit is to take a fresh fig, mash it with a spoon, and smear the resulting jam on fresh whole wheat bread. For those of you who aren't able to grow your own, you can make a similar spread out of the dried fruit. Simmer four cups of dried figs in four cups of water until the figs fall apart and mash easily. Finish the mashing process with a wire whisk and put the fig spread in the fridge in a covered jar. Figs are so good for you that you never have to feel guilty about spreading fig jam on your bread.

As for the cancer facts I mentioned earlier, scientists at the Institute of Physical and Chemical Research at the Mitsubishi-Kasei Institute of Life Sciences in Tokyo discovered a chemical contained in the fig that does indeed treat the disease. When the Japanese implanted cancer cells into mice and then injected the sites with fig extracts, the tumors shrank down by a third. The substance benzal-

Fig 49

dehyde was then tested on other cancer patients with wonderful success. It seems Isaiah knew what he was doing.

Today, the closest most of us come to the fruit is in a Fig Newton, and if this is how you get your saving dose, more power to you. There is no bad way to consume the fruit, and with this one's track record, we should all make it a daily routine. The really exciting part is that a fresh fig is the most wonderful fruit in the world. If you haven't tasted a fig fresh from the tree, and I mean one you grew yourself, you have missed one of the greatest pleasures in life. The moment the fig hits your tongue, your head says that this is ambrosia, the food of the gods. Even fresh ones at the market don't compare, as the fig gets its sugar in the last days on the tree, and the fresh ones you can buy in the store are picked before they are ripe, which in my mind defeats the point.

So grow them yourself. I was told when I moved to Washington, D.C., that it was too cold to grow figs, and I now have 250 different varieties thriving in my backyard. If you live north of the Mason-Dixon line, plant the fig in a pot and bring it into the basement for the winter. You can start your own fig tree with a branch of somebody else's, or order a rooted tree from one of the many mail-order houses that deal in them.

▼▼▼▼▼▼▼▼▼▼▼▼▼▼▼▼▼▼▼▼▼

GARLIC
Allium sativum

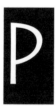erhaps the most universally accepted panacea known to man, garlic is one home remedy that has been proven effective. An Egyptian medical papyrus dating from around 1500 B.C. lists 22 garlic prescriptions for such complaints as headaches and throat disorders, and the slaves who built the Great Pyramids at Giza, for whom being sick was not an option, are said to have eaten piles of garlic for strength. And I do mean piles. In World War I, garlic was used to fight typhus and dysentery; in World War II, British physicians treating battle wounds with garlic reported total success in warding off septic poisoning and gangrene.

Garlic was once known as poor man's treacle, or heal-all, as it cured just about whatever ailed you—that seems to have been, and still to be, the case. The

Arabs, who believe that garlic grew from the footprint of Satan as he stepped out of the Garden of Eden, have so many uses for the plant that it's hard to enumerate them. Ditto the Chinese and Indians. Garlic's medicinal value is not subject to debate, it is a reality. Garlic could save your life on a number of scores. You should eat it, and you should eat it on a regular basis. And that's about all there is to it.

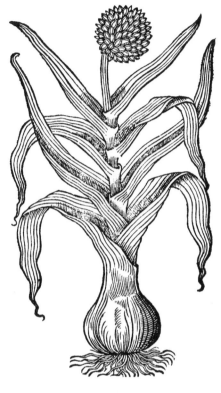

The garlic we buy in our supermarkets grows wild in the Near East and has for centuries, although no one knows exactly where it originated. The ancient Israelites were familiar with 67 kinds of onions and garlic, and the Crusaders who ran into the plant in their effort to take back the Holy Land reputedly did take a bit of it back with them to Europe in the form of the odorous bulb.

There it found numerous uses, perhaps the most curious being as a safeguard for grave robbers. It seems that when people died of the plague, they were buried with their jewels on. Even the greediest of relatives was unwilling to remove baubles from an infected body. The thieves of the day found this custom a bit too tempting, and a sect developed that ravaged the mass graves of plague victims. They did this with not a care in the world. Why? Because they washed themselves, their clothes, and the jewelry with garlic vinegar. Garlic's scientifically proven germ-killing qualities did the trick on the rings and bracelets—great insurance for a high-risk, high-return profession—and the thieves made a bundle.

Throughout history, garlic has been used internationally to treat lung problems from pneumonia to bronchitis. The fact that it does contain chemicals which kill bacteria may partially explain its effective use in this vein. Somehow though, its powers go beyond the logical, and the plant, whether eaten hot or made into cough syrup, definitely speeds the healing process of a cold, which is something we'd all like to do.

The Shakers were garlic's biggest fans in the lung department. In the late 1800s, their communities used the smelly plant to treat all related conditions most effectively. Remember, these were the folks who made healing a way of life and a profession. They did not offer things for sale that did not work.

For those with a taste for alcohol, the traditional West Virginia cure for asthma and other lung ailments is garlic soaked in gin. The juniper berries used to flavor the gin would also shore up the ailing, as you will see on page 73, but what the flavor would be like, I cannot attest.

GARLIC. In days gone by, garlic was seen primarily as a food, not a flavoring, and more than one ancient dinner consisted of roasted garlic on toast, my own favorite. Roast five or six bulbs of garlic on a baking tin in the oven at 400° for 45 minutes. When they're done, they scream to be smeared on a good cracker. Peel the outer skin off the meat, and go to it. They're great as is, but I also learned from a gypsy in Spain that the roasted cloves bathed in a light vinaigrette of olive oil, red pepper, salt, and a touch of lemon juice make one of the best spreads around.

Past and present root doctors in the Louisiana bayou recommend garlic when you have "live things jumping around in your stomach." To be blunt, we are talking about worms, amoebas, and other little items that take up residence in the gut. At one time, the cure was to boil a silver coin with a lady on one side and nine pieces of garlic in one cup of milk, then drink the milk on an empty stomach. The root doctors also suggested wearing garlic and asafoetida around the neck to prevent picking up the epidemic disease du jour, and they specified that when you're using garlic for epidemic, you shouldn't ask for it—it should be given without solicitation.

Apparently when a disease swept through the neighborhood, as it was apt to do in that moist, swampy region, the custom was for neighbors to go from house to house, offering their friends and relations garlic to keep them safe from pestilence. A piece of garlic wrapped in cotton and inserted into the ear was thought to cure earaches. As garlic does contain a natural bacteria killer, placing some in an infected ear would, in fact, kill the bacteria causing the pain. Garlic ground with animal fat was the leading antiseptic ointment for cuts.

My great-grandmother, adhering to the Israelite tradition of garlic as a Jewish cure-all, always kept a pot of garlic boiling in her backyard to treat her high blood pressure. This country belief was seconded by an informant in Utah. It seems that Brigham Young, when traveling west, made sure he and his packed a lot of garlic, and some of his followers are still using it to this day. Boiled garlic is eaten hot to kick out a cold that won't go away, and eating raw garlic is believed to make your blood unappealing to mosquitoes.

Residents of the Tennessee mountains traditionally collected wild garlic as a spring tonic to kill off any lingering winter illnesses. The wild garlic, *Allium vineale*, is presumed to have many of the same active properties as the Near Eastern version. In rural North Carolina, garlic was beaten and eaten for boils and pneumonia. The Pennsylvania Dutch also used wild garlic, which they call *wilder knowwelloch*, to bring boils and ulcers to a head, but they put it directly on the eruption. Inflamed bowels were treated by applying a mash of wild garlic and bran to the stomach, and a tea made of the same was used as a liver tonic.

The National Library of Medicine, in Bethesda, Maryland, a marvelous and prestigious collection of medical literature, contains about 125 scientific papers on garlic published since 1983. Studies of garlic reveal potent compounds that appear to retard heart disease, stroke, cancer, and a wide range of infections. Let's take a gander at what has panned out about garlic.

For one thing, garlic indeed kills bacteria. A chemical contained in the bulb, allicin, is said to be even stronger than penicillin and tetracycline. Allicin's claim to fame is that it is a broad-spectrum bug killer, and gets rid of most of the nasty beasts that make us lose a day of work. The bad news is that allicin is the smelly part of the bulb—no smell, no antibiotic. Garlic also lowers blood cholesterol, thins the blood, and lowers blood pressure, the three factors that cause heart disease.

Garlic acts as a strong expectorant and decongestant for the lungs as well. People suffering from chronic bronchitis are greatly helped by adding this plant to their diets. What's more, animals fed on garlic don't develop cancerous tumors, and human beings who eat garlic are less likely to get cancer than those who don't.

The down side of including this one in our tonic is that it isn't going to do much for the flavor, but based on garlic's reputation, how could you leave it out? And we're not talking about garlic powder, we're talking about the freshly ground item. Hey, it's for your health.

GINGER

Zingiber officinale

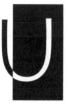

ntil recently, the only ginger North Americans knew was the ground variety on their spice racks. Today you can buy hands of ginger in the produce department of almost any grocery store. These "hands" or roots are actually rhizomes or underground stems. Bite into a fresh ginger root, and you will feel the sun's fire stored in the papery brown wrapper.

The ginger we're most familiar with is *Zingiber officinale*, the official ginger, but the family is much more extensive and includes cardamom, tumeric, and zedoary. In Asia, where the reedlike plant originated, all members are thought good for preserving health, and *Zingiber officinale* is considered a general tonic. It keeps you from losing your health in the first place, and helps you to find it if you have misplaced it.

Ginger was well known to the ancients. The Greeks and Romans, who considered it an Arabian product because, along with other spices from India, it came to them by way of the Red Sea, used it extensively. It was a common article of import from the East to Europe by the 11th century A.D. The Europeans, like people worldwide, prized it as both a spice and a domestic remedy.

Ginger made its way to tropical America early in the colonial era. Today the invasive plant grows there in abundance, and the locals gather it for just about any malady. The pungent fresh rhizomes are sold by herb vendors in Caracas, Venezuela, where they are pounded to a paste to be applied to the abdomen in case of difficult menstruation. In Costa Rica, merchants declare that a ginger decoction will relieve throat inflammation and asthma. With honey added, it is a valued remedy for bronchitis and coughs, and it also serves as a sudorific in fevers. One Panamanian herb seller said that she had a special variety to relieve rheumatism. Guatemalans take ginger decoctions as a stomachic and tonic. In Trinidad, it's a remedy for indigestion, stomachache, and malaria, and the fumes from an infusion in urine are inhaled to relieve head colds.

The Arabs use two other members of the same family, galanga (*Alpinia officinarum*) and zedoary (*Curcuma zedoaria*), for treatment of stomach ailments and for general wellness. The roots of these two plants are also considered to be stimulants, aphrodisiacs, and of all things, cures for amnesia. Pounded with olive oil, they are added to a hot bath or rubbed onto the body for any form of muscle complaint due to overexertion. In North Africa, this usually comes from plowing, but the treatment would be as good for someone who has worked out too strenuously at the gym. Ginger is also especially recommended for muscle complaints due to age; its oil is massaged into the affected parts for rheumatism and arthritic conditions.

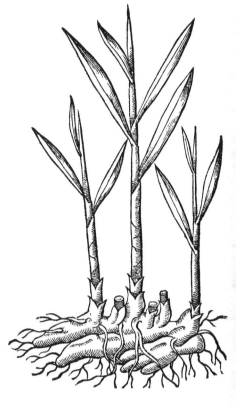

To increase strength and vigor, ground roots mixed with honey are taken in the morning. The Arabs find that this tonic is especially good for those suffering from weakness in the lungs and genitals. For the aphrodisiac effect, the root is combined with black pepper; for lung deficiencies of any sort, the root is combined with honey, cloves, and olive oil. The same mixture is used in the case of poisonous animal bites.

In China, where the science of ginger is so exacting that gingers from different parts of the country are used for different purposes—some for cooking, some for illness; some dry, some fresh—fresh ginger is used to cure coughs, nausea, gas, and dysentery. A stomach stimulant, it's also used to treat fevers and mushroom poisoning, which is a particularly nasty piece of business. Certain varieties of mushrooms contain many highly toxic chemicals, and when the liver tries to get these out of the blood stream, the liver itself is destroyed in the process. As we all know, when the liver goes, wave good-bye. This use ties in with the reputation of several ginger relatives as cures for hangovers, which are partly caused by the severe beating the liver takes when people overdo with alcohol.

The ground ginger with which we are most acquainted is thought to have originated in Mongolia, and its name in the Chinese dialects indicates this. It is now grown in all provinces of China. Despite its Chinese roots, the dry ginger we get at the grocery store comes from Jamaica and parts of Africa. This is because ground ginger only contains the meat of the rhizome, and the Chinese ginger doesn't separate from the skin as readily as its Jamaican counterpart.

In China, dried ginger is used for all the things that fresh ginger is in addition to hemorrhages, perverted lochia, constipation, and urinary difficulties. Ginger gets the kidneys working and helps flush out the system. Of this I know. Once in the aim of avoiding a cold, I drank ginger tea for several days. I couldn't figure out why I kept running to the rest room; some time later, I discovered that ginger is a natural diuretic.

In India, we find ginger used to treat chronic rheumatism: the patient takes an infusion of ginger before going to bed and is then covered heavily with blankets to encourage copious perspiration. The same treatment is also considered beneficial in cases of colds or catarrhal attacks and during the cold stage of an intermittent fever. People plagued with embarrassing gas take ginger with salt before meals. Ginger is also said to clean the tongue and throat, increase the appetite, and produce an agreeable sensation. The profuse flow of saliva that comes from chewing a piece of ginger root is considered beneficial to those suffering from sore throats, hoarseness, and loss of voice.

GINGER. A number of years ago a Jamaican friend suggested an island use for ginger that has stuck with me ever since. Take fresh ginger from the garden or the grocery, lay it out on a piece of newspaper, and flatten it with a hammer. Place one cup of the flattened, unpeeled root in a gallon of water and bring the mixture to a rolling boil. Take it off the heat, strain the ginger shards from it, and add sugar or honey to taste. The mixture can be drunk like that or put into a carbonizer (available at any bar supply store) for a real treat—homemade ginger ale.

On the scientific level, almost all of the folk beliefs have been verified. Ginger prevents motion sickness, thins the blood, elevates the blood pressure, lowers blood cholesterol, and prevents cancer in animals. Ginger extracts are reported to exhibit numerous pharmacological properties, among them stimulating the vasomotor and respiratory centers as well as the hearts of anesthetized cats. The extracts also lower serum and hepatic cholesterol in rats previously fed cholesterol and kill vaginal trichomonads in vitro. Chinese researchers have reported that fresh ginger is highly effective in the clinical treatment of rheumatism, acute bacterial dysentery, malaria, and inflammation of the testicles.

As for its effects on the gastrointestinal system, tests on dogs indicate that doses of 0.1 to 1.0 gram result in an increase in the secretion of gastric juice.

Animals fed ginger at the same time as chemicals that normally induce vomiting did not throw up.

Suffice it to say, if your stomach is upset, a glass of fresh ginger tea will settle it. Around the globe, people prevent praying to the porcelain god with ginger.

▼▼▼▼▼▼▼▼▼▼▼▼▼▼▼▼▼▼▼▼

GINSENG
Panax quinquefolium

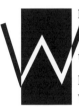

hen I sat down to write this section on ginseng, I did so with apprehension, mostly due to the huge pile of papers I'd accumulated on the subject: it is perhaps the most-written-about and best-known tonic plant in the world. Still, despite its phenomenal reputation, many Westerners who have used ginseng say that it doesn't work. And from the perspective of someone accustomed to Western medicine, they're right. Ginseng doesn't speed you up, slow you down, make you nervous, or do anything else that is immediately detectable. If you're looking for something that carries the nerve damage of medicines that make you "feel funny," look elsewhere.

This is in part the problem many Westerners have with herbal medicine: herbs simply do not pack the sensory punch we're used to. All of our major cough medications contain an incredible amount of alcohol. I know this because I don't take alcohol under any circumstance, and one of the reasons I investigated herbal medicines in the first place was that I could not find an alcohol-free cough syrup. All of our cold medications come with substances that make us feel different, and really different at that. If a medication doesn't make us feel medicated in half an hour, we ask for something else.

To talk about ginseng, we need to acknowledge our tendency to think that effective medication has to instantly change the way we feel. Ginseng is not a drugging agent, but it does work. It helps the body, and in the long haul, it could save our lives.

Ginseng's biggest champions, the Chinese, have been searching their own lands and their neighbors' for more than 2,000 years to satisfy their desire for the powerful, rare, and accordingly, costly plant. To them, it is the supreme tonic for both the treatment and the prevention of all illnesses. Incredible longevity comes along with its daily use. At some point in time, every culture in the world has looked for the fountain of youth. The Chinese feel they have found it in ginseng.

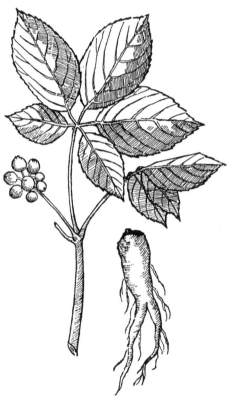

Inspired both by its power and by the unusual, vaguely human shape of its roots, countless myths surround the plant. One belief is that ginseng forms when lightning strikes the earth, and as such, it contains all the energy previously possessed by the lightning bolt, energy which is then conveyed to the eater. Perhaps the most colorful Chinese legend holds that over time the root of the ginseng develops an increasingly manlike form, and after 300 years, the root gets up and walks away from its spot in the ground. Though this being can pass for human, its blood is white rather than red; if the creature can be caught, its blood is so healing that it can resuscitate a dead man. But the capture has to happen soon after the root-man leaves the earth, as he is star-bound, on his way to live among the constellations.

Whether you believe ginseng can get up and take a walk or not, there is something special about the plant that does not yield to rational explanation. Throughout their history, the Chinese have more than believed in ginseng, they have raped the land, tortured and killed people—you name it, they have done it—to get their hands on the substance, and in the early 18th century, the insatiable demand spread from Asia to the Americas.

North American native ginseng first came to the attention of Europeans when Father Joseph Lafitau, who had been a missionary in China, identified the similar North American plant growing near a Mohawk village in Canada in 1716.

Lafitau learned of the plant from a Father Jartoux, who two years earlier had written *A Description of a Tartarian Plant Called Ginseng*. In this work, Jartoux detailed his personal experiences with the plant while in China and correctly predicted the discovery of ginseng in North America, based upon a comparison of the climates of China and Canada. Jartoux set up ovens for curing the roots, and had the Mohawks gather and process them for the Chinese market. By 1717, it was being brought from as far away as Green Bay, Wisconsin, by the Fox Indians, and shipped to Hong Kong via France.

The trade quickly prospered. In 1752, a shipment of spoiled roots so shattered the faith of the Asian buyers that it took nearly a century for the market to fully recover. Still, the high demand threatened to eradicate what was always a rare plant. By 1798, John Drayton of South Carolina said of ginseng, "It is so much sought after by the Cherokees for trade, it is by no means as plentiful as it used to be in this state." Ginseng gathering had begun to be a way of life for many pioneers. A man could go "sang hunting" and return with a fortune, or, in those perilous times, never return at all.

Both the Native Americans and the early colonists who gathered the roots for trade also used ginseng for a variety of medicinal purposes themselves. The colonists made it into tea to encourage the appetite or strengthen the digestion, particularly of elderly persons or puny children. Ginseng plus black cherry and yellowroot made a potent tonic, especially with the addition of some homemade whiskey, and an early herbal suggested gathering ginseng root and steeping it with chamomile flowers for fainting females. Colonel William Byrd, in his *History of the Dividing Line*, wrote:

To help cure fatigue, I used to chew a root of ginseng as I walked along. This kept up my spirits. It gives an uncommon warmth and vigor to the blood. It cheers the heart of a man that has a bad wife, and makes him look down with great composure upon the crosses of the world. It will make old age amiable by rendering it lively, cheerful, and good humored.

By 1800, several patent medicines on the market featured "seng" or "sang-tone," and between 1889 and 1905, ginseng farms popped up all over the United States, with centers in Amberg, Wisconsin, and Chardon, Ohio. Ironically, the United States buys ginseng products from Asia that are made with roots raised in America and shipped abroad for processing.

Few medicinal plants have been more widely or thoroughly researched than ginseng. One recent study shows that ginseng seems to do the work of the hormones which the adrenal cortex naturally produces in response to everyday stress.

As a result, the body does not have to manufacture them in such large amounts, and the adrenal cortex does not become overworked.

In addition to sex hormones, the adrenal glands manufacture hormones that regulate sugar metabolism and hormones that regulate the mineral content of body tissues. Adaptive as it is, this vital organ was not designed to work well under conditions of frequent or prolonged stress. These are the conditions of modern life, and they can lead to a number of diverse symptoms, including high blood pressure, heart disease, ulcers, anxiety, and chronic fatigue. A variety of tests on animals confirm that ginseng plays a positive role in combatting stress.

GINSENG. You may be surprised to discover that when boiled into a tea, ginseng tastes rather like dirt. Folks certainly haven't been using it for centuries for its flavor! The roots are sold whole or in a processed, hardened red mass of slices. I find the slices more convenient; as a single person I rarely need as much tea as a whole root produces. To make tea, place three slices in a cup and a half of boiling water, let the water boil down to one cup, strain the liquid, and drink it sweetened with something, anything, please!

In one experiment, chickens were exposed to extreme cold over a two-month period. This normally tends to decrease their egg-laying capacity, but the hens that received daily doses of ginseng continued to produce as usual, laying over twice as many eggs as the control group.

In another experiment, mice were made to run on an inclined moving ramp. The mice treated with extracts of ginseng for 12 days prior to the test were able to run on the ramp 50 percent longer than the untreated group.

Laboratory rats that were not treated with ginseng lived an average of about 659 days; those that were given ginseng lived an average of about 768 days. Similar tests have not yet been performed on humans, but the equivalent of this difference would amount to an extension of the average life span by about ten years. I would settle for ten extra years.

An anabolic is a substance that builds up the general health of the body by regulating the burning of energy. The opposite of an anabolic is a catabolic (the drug amphetamine is a good example). It temporarily gives a person more energy, but does so by tearing down the body's energy reserves. In a sense, one process is healthy and constructive, the other process is unhealthy and can be destructive if it is continued for a long period of time. The steroid constituents of ginseng are so similar in their structure to the body's own anabolic agents that it is certainly very feasible that they act in a similar manner.

In addition to its steroid components, ginseng also contains vitamins B1 and B2, calcium, potassium, iron, sodium, silicon, magnesium, titanium, barium, strontium, aluminum, manganese, sugar, starch, mucilage, and a number of substances that are unique to the plant. These include panasen, which some researchers believe has a direct stimulant effect on the brain similar to that of caffeine; ginsenin, which somewhat resembles insulin in its effects and probably explains the beneficial effect of ginseng in the treatment of alloxan diabetes; and panoxic acid, which facilitates the efficient functioning of the cardiovascular system, helps prevent the formation of cholesterol, and is thought to facilitate burning of the body's fat deposits. Also present are panaxin, a substance that directly stimulates the central nervous system and acts as a tonic to the heart and circulatory system, and panaquilon, a substance believed to stimulate the endocrine system in general and to maintain proper hormone levels in the body.

The literature on ginseng's healthful benefits is voluminous. Its anti-stress capabilities are well documented. For our purposes, though, perhaps the most important thing to realize is that due to its anabolic nature, ginseng acts in a manner that may not be noticeable at first. Give it time. Regular users of ginseng report that they are less tired at the end of a hard week. Many people with busy, hectic schedules say that they feel less tension under pressure and have more energy left over to do the things they want to do. And that's something all of us could use.

▼▼▼▼▼▼▼▼▼▼▼▼▼▼▼▼▼▼▼▼▼▼▼▼

GRAPE
Vitis vinifera

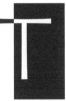here is a long-held notion among practitioners of herbal medicine that when we consume a plant, we consume its very nature. In ancient and not-so-ancient times, the recommendation has been that when we are weak, we should eat strong plants, and the grape is one strong plant.

Have you ever seen a grapevine growing? It's nothing short of incredible. Plants disclose their power if you learn to look for it. And when you see a massive grapevine, 40 feet long, covered with 200 pounds of ripe grapes swinging with sugar perfection, you know there is something special about this plant.

The grape is thought to be one of the oldest plants in continuous cultivation, and written records of it date back to the days of Noah, 2300 B.C. In addition to its more familiar byproducts, the grape provided the early Israelites with dibs, an ancient food item once found in every home. Dibs was made by boiling freshly squeezed grape juice down to reduce its water content until there was nothing

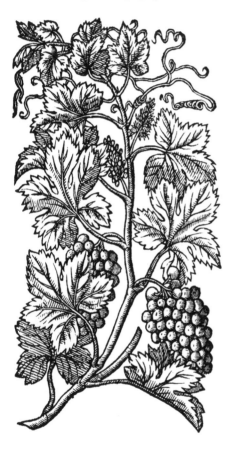

left but the sugary essence of the grape. The substance was so high in sugar that it did not spoil, and it was used much as we now use grape jelly. Unlike grape products today, however, dibs was considered a powerful health giver.

The fruit's Chinese name, *pu tao*, indicates that it is not a native plant, but rather one that came from afar. Though no one knows when the grape reached China, it has been in use there for at least 2,000 years. The Chinese find the fruit, root, stem, leaf, and other by-products strengthening to the body. For those whose health is threatened, the grape is called in to shore up things. The fermented product, commonly called wine, is said by the Chinese to prevent hunger, stimulate the instinct, and quiet the mind. I could have told you that.

From our 17th-century European herbalist friend Gerard, we hear "that raisins chewed with pepper draw flegme and water out of the head," and "they be moreover a remedy for the inflammation of the mouth, and almonds of the throat, if they be gargled, or the mouth washed therewith." He also noted that an application of grapevine sap would "taketh away superfluous hairs," and declared, in case it's a problem in your family, that the grape "stayeth the lusting or longing of women with child, though they be but outwardly applied, and also taken inwardly any manner of ways."

Galen went on to "affirmeth":

Thirty Plants That Can Save Your Life!

There is in the sweet ones a temperate and smoothing quality, with a power to cleanse moderately. They are good for the chest, lungs, windpipe, kidneys, bladder, and for the stomach; for they make smooth the roughness of the windpipe, and are good against hoarseness, shortness of breath, or difficulty of breathing: they serve to concoct the spittle, and to cause it to rise more easily in any disease whatsoever of the chest, sides, and lungs, and do mitigate the pain of the kidneys and bladder, which hath joined with it heat and sharpness of urine: they dull and allay the malice of sharpe and biting humors that hurt the mouth of the stomach.

Although colonials arrived in the New World with grapevines in hand, the Native Americans were already quite familiar with a native variety. The Creek Indians used a concoction of boiled grape shoots and tendrils to speed the recovery of snakebite victims. The Seminoles had a variety of uses for the native grape, *Vitis palmatto*, which they called *palko lakko*; perhaps the most important of these was their treatment for diabetics: four doses a day of tea made from the entire plant. Like the Creek snakebite cure, this suggests that the grape may assist the all-important function of the liver.

An unfaithful spouse is definitely threatening to the health—not necessarily yours, but somebody's. The Seminoles believed that if you took a grape tendril, wrapped a lock of your spouse's hair around it, and buried it at the door stoop, it would keep him or her from stepping out.

The Seminoles also used the plant to keep their hair from falling out, and the Delawares said that grapes could make hair grow as long as the vines themselves. They tapped the vines in early spring, collected the sap, and used it as a shampoo to make their hair shiny and lush. Scalp conditions of all sorts were treated with this sap and with a tea made of the bark. Of course, Gerard said that grape sap *removed* hair, so I would definitely do a test patch before using it myself.

A Dr. A. M. Liebstein writing in 1927 didn't have anything to say about unwanted body hair or randy spouses, pregnant or otherwise, but in general, he agreed with his predecessors:

GRAPE. In addition to eating fresh grapes or drinking them in the form of wine or juice, you can also try my recipe for a tasty grape syrup. Take four pounds of fresh grapes (red or white), three tablespoons of freshly grated ginger, two cups of dried sorrel blossoms, and four cups of water, put them in a pot, and simmer on low until the grapes have fallen apart. Allow the mixture to cool. Hold a new pair of panty hose over a bowl, pour the mixture into one of the legs, and allow the swollen leg to hang until the liquid has dripped into the bowl. When you want a drink that is really different, add two tablespoons of this syrup and some ice to a tumbler of club soda, sit back, and get healthy.

Grapes next to apples have been crowned the queen of fruits. Grapes are good for all dyspeptic conditions, febrile conditions, liver and kidney troubles, tuberculosis of the lungs and bones, hemorrhoids, varicose veins, osteomyelitis, gangrene, cancer, a great many other malignant diseases.

Obviously the good doctor was a big fan of the grape. Let's follow up on some of his claims for the grape as a healthful substance.

Grapes contain tannins based on polyphenols, which make them antiviral, antitumor, antibacterial, and antifungal. As bacteria, virus, and tumors are responsible for many of the modern medical woes, this is exciting news! In recent scientific research the grape has been proven to be antiviral against both the polio virus and the herpes simplex virus in a test tube. Researchers Konowalchuk and Speirs in Canada tested grape products available at the supermarket against a host of micro-organisms. The overriding conclusion was that grapes in fact act against many disease-causing organisms. Maybe the old adage should be revised to say, "A grape a day keeps the doctor away."

Tannins are complex substances produced by the life processes of most higher plants; some produce a lot of tannins, some less. Tannins's antimicrobial powers are well documented. Unfortunately, most plant tannins are not absorbed into the blood stream. They pass right out of the gut without entering the blood vessels that line it. Interestingly enough, the tannins contained in the grape are absorbed into the blood in the digestive process. Once in the blood, tannins could move through the blood stream knocking out bacteria, virus, and developing cancers.

Moreover, grapes have a high amount of caffeic acid in their succulent and dried flesh. This acid has been shown to prevent cancer growth in animals. In folk medicine grapes have long been used to prevent cancer and treat people with cancer.

The grape and all its by-products were highly rated by the ancients; its continual mention in the Bible testifies to this fact. Remember, the Bible is an agricultural as well as a sacred text, filled with observations made from centuries of trial and error. If it was good enough for the patriarchs and matriarchs, it's good enough for me.

HONEY
Miel

Our next ingredient isn't really a plant—it's a plant by-product—but as one of the world's most medicinal and universally used plant products, it makes a perfect addition to the tonic pot. As ignorant as we are about plants as curative agents, most of us do know that lemon and honey will sooth a sore throat about as well as anything. But there's more to honey's age-old role as healer.

I have kept my innate desire to tell personal stories to a minimum in this book, but I will allow myself this one. When I was in northern Spain researching herbal plants, I came across a honey seller whose shop offered more than 20 different kinds. The honeys were classified according to what plants they were collected from, and next to each type of honey was a placard listing its medicinal value—the honey collected from sage plants was used for bronchial infections, the honey collected from thyme for bladder infections and weaknesses, and so on. Not only did I not know so many different honeys existed, I also didn't know that each honey had a very different medicinal purpose. I had never thought beyond clover honey in plastic bear-shaped bottles "for your convenience." I knew that honey was made by bees and at least couldn't be bad for you, but that was all. I had no idea that the world of honey was so complex, and my time with the friendly honey seller sparked an interest which I plan to share with you now. Get ready for some information on the next plant that could save your life.

Let's start with what honey is. I was under the impression that bees made honey, but this is inaccurate. Plants make nectar; bees collect and process nectar into honey. Plants produce nectar in nectaries, which are glands located in the center of the flower. These nectaries pump out liquid sugars made in the leaves. The nectar-collecting bees hook themselves up to these sugar pumps and fill their stomachs with the sweet liquid. They then fly to the hive where they regurgitate the nectar into the empty cells of the honey comb. A different class of bees then sit on the combs and fan them to evaporate the water contained in the nectar. When the nectar has evaporated down to one quarter of its original water content, yet another class of bees produce wax and seal the cells with it.

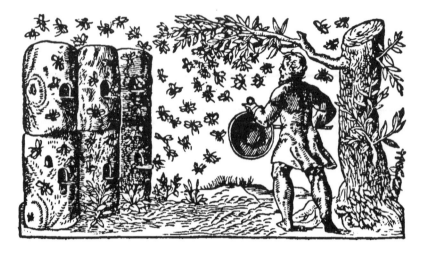

When you eat honey, you are really eating the nectar of flowers, which is essentially a captured form of the sun's power. Along with the sugars produced in the leaves, honey contains other ingredients characteristic of individual plant species. This accounts for the different sorts of honeys out there—tulip poplar honey is dark, and clover honey is light; orange blossom honey smells of orange blossoms; and honey collected from garlic blossoms initially has a garlicky taste. So on top of having the power of the sun, honey holds powers specific to the plant from which it was collected. Thus, it makes sense that different honeys have different health characteristics.

Bees are kept for honey collection from the North to the South Poles, wherever man lives and flowers bloom. Unlike other animals kept in captivity, bees have not changed an iota in all the millions of years human beings have kept them for the sweet, healing product they produce. There is no such thing as a tame bee; they all come with the equipment needed to do battle with our sensitive skin, a situation which, from the human point of view, has not improved since the cave days when beekeeping started.

Prehistoric cave paintings in both Switzerland and Spain depict men hanging on cliffs to take honey from beehives. The painting from Spain shows a man with his hand in the hive, snatching honey while out-of-scale bees swarm around him. As a beekeeper, I would draw the experience the same way. Those little insects seem pretty large when they're crawling all over you!

The earliest written records indicate that 4,000 years before Christ, the

Egyptians were loading hives on boats and sailing up the Nile until they came to the places far to the south where flowers were beginning to bloom. As is obvious from the large number of papyrus scrolls and hieroglyphic tablets which deal with beekeeping, the Egyptians were keen on honey. The bee was their symbol of power and health, and they used it on jewelry, pottery, art, and architecture. The pharaoh even had a bee stamp which he placed right next to his signature on official documents.

Egyptian doctors saw honey as the ultimate healing substance, and it was one of the most important materials used in religious rites. Lovers exchanged honey pots as symbols of their eternal devotion, and bridegrooms had to agree to give their brides a specified amount of honey every single year according to the woman's social ranking.

Royal families customarily were buried with large quantities of honey to prepare them in style for the afterlife, and the pharaoh went to his eternal rest with enough honey to keep several villages healthy for a century. When Queen Tiy's parents' tomb was excavated and a jar of honey was found, the honey was still in good shape after more than 3,000 years.

Which brings up one of the strangest honey facts: it never goes bad. Nobody knows how bees do it, but bacteria cannot grow in honey. This was one of the reasons why bomb shelters during World War II were stocked with honey and wheat germ: people could survive on nothing but those two substances for long periods of time, and their food supply would never have spoiled however long they were down there.

Like the Egyptians, the ancient Greeks and Romans were fond of honey, which they felt helped make the mind and the body more vital and strong. Roman gladiators, who understandably enough took their life-and-death profession pretty seriously, were fed as much honey as they could eat, and Greek bees still produce some of the best honey in the world, collected from wild mountain thyme and oregano.

During the Middle Ages in Europe, straw hives were often kept on the walls

HONEY. A few years back, I developed allergies, mostly to plants. This was an unpleasant development for a person who lives and breathes plants day in and day out. In seeking out relief, I found research that showed eating honey from your immediate vicinity relieves allergies. I decided to give it a try. I take one tablespoon every morning in the hope of losing my allergies, and I believe it has worked. Many of the long-lived persons I have met around the world feel that a teaspoon of honey a day, whether in tea, on toast, or straight, is one factor in their extended and healthy lives.

of fortified cities. From there, the bees could collect honey in the surrounding countryside, and in case of an attack, the city's defenders could easily hurl the hives down on the attackers' heads. Talk about a home security system! These were the excitable black bees of northern Europe, and once an armor-clad knight had a dozen or so inside the visor of his helmet (and they would go right for those dark slits), I imagine he would be pretty preoccupied until he got them out again.

Throughout history, people who didn't intend to use their bees for stinging the crap out of their enemies have still gone to considerable trouble to secure a ready supply of honey. Of course, they kept bees because the honey tasted good, but they also kept them because honey was considered one of the single most healthful items they could have around the house.

This point was driven home to me in northern Spain when I met a man named Hanibal in an apple orchard way up in the mountains of Asturias. He was working on a new wall, lugging stones and breaking them with a single stroke of a not-so-small hammer. In conversation, I learned that he was the age of my grandfather, a man who has a hard time getting out of his chair. I asked the Spaniard what he ate, and he responded, "Honey every day." He would be the first of many elderly persons I encountered there who were still running around like spring chickens. They all told me that honey was the key to staying healthy and vital well into old age.

I have been told by more than one know-it-all that honey is just sugar, which is partly true and also totally inaccurate. First of all, it comes packing the essence of whatever plant originally produced it, but beyond this, it is different from the cane sugar that comes in a bag. Composed of the same sugars contained in fruit, dextrose and levulose, honey does not require the complex digestive process that cane sugar does. Honey is an inverted sugar—that is to say it is already partially digested and can enter the body as energy instantly. Cane sugar is sucrose. It will kill a diabetic; honey will not.

Hanibal suggested that if I ate honey every day for a month, I would have more energy, and he was right. Honey has been used to preserve health and to treat every condition that man has ever suffered. The list is too long to even bother including, but most recently honey has found use in treating allergies, a condition that can certainly ruin your quality of life. Many cultures have considered honey a miracle food for one simple reason: it is. No one understands exactly why this is so, but I think that this isn't as important as knowing that honey is one food we should all eat regularly.

▼▼▼▼▼▼▼▼▼▼▼▼▼▼▼▼▼▼▼▼▼▼

JUJUBE
Ziziphus jujuba

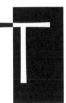

hat's right, jujubes could save your life. In fairness, I must tell you that the jujube I am referring to is not the confection sold at the dime store and movie house. It's the genuine item, a life-giving and restoring sweet treat few Westerners have ever had the pleasure of tasting. The real jujube fruit is the product of an Asian tree, *Jujube ziziphus*. It looks like an olive, but tastes like an apple in both its dried and fresh forms. It is a preferred fruit of the Orient for health and table eating. Whereas we Westerners say that an apple a day keeps the doctor away, the Asians believe that a jujube does the same trick.

These dried fruits made their way from Asia into Europe during the days of Marco Polo. Sometimes called Chinese dates, they're slightly less sugary than actual dates, and they found such favor in Europe that in time the term *jujube* came to apply to any dried sweetmeat and then to candy in general. Though the candies sold at theaters today probably have no natural ingredients at all, their namesake is quite natural, and healthy as well.

Despite its unfamiliarity to most Westerners, the jujube is known from Arabia to the far reaches of the Orient. The main jujube is called *Ziziphus jujube*, but other members of the same tribe—*Z. ziziphus* and *Z. spina-christi*—all find medicinal use. The Arabs, who use the fruit of all three trees to ensure health, feel that the leaves of the plant kill parasites and worms in the intestinal tract which cause diarrhea. The fruits are said to cure coughs, resolve any other lung complaints, soothe the internal organs, and, last but not least, reduce water retention.

In Haiti, twelve fruits or a handful of leaves and roots are boiled in several cups of water to make a tea taken as an antidote to poison. I've said it before, but the modern world is filled with poison, most of which we take into our bodies without any coaxing, and the jujube may be the corrective we need.

To learn more about the jujube, it is best to go to its home, Asia, where the fruit has been cultivated since ancient days. The Asians use two kinds of jujubes, a wild sort and a domestic type. Although the two are closely related, there are some important differences, the first noteworthy one being that the spines have been bred out of the domestic plant, making picking easier.

The wild plant is called *suan-tsao*. As you may have noticed earlier, one of the medicinal jujubes I've mentioned is called *Ziziphus spina-christi*, and you guessed it, the name means Christ's spiny jujube. That plant gets a whopping seven listings in the Bible, including one rather unpleasant quotation from the Book of Judges: "Then I will tear your flesh with the thorns of the wilderness, and with briars." It's no exaggeration. Some jujubes, like the wild Asian *suan-zao*, make a good old southern bramble patch seem like a bed of silk. *Suan-zao* produces a small, sour fruit that is used mainly for the stomach and as a general tonic.

The Chinese have found that the wild jujube fruit improves the health of the body. In fact, the common belief is that if the fruit is taken on a daily basis, it will improve skin color and tone, both signs of physical well-being. The tree, by the way, is said to have been discovered by a fairy or angel-like creature who disclosed it to humanity for our benefit.

Its domestic counterpart, known as *pei-tsao* in northern China and *nan-tsao* in the south, is considered to be cooling to the body. Like an Asian version of the aspirin, the fruits somehow reduce pain and distress. They are strongly recommended for cases of sleeplessness caused from mental fatigue, physical weakness, or pain. They reign supreme in the treatment of rheumatic symptoms and are said to rejuvenate the body, whether it is suffering from stress or age. The plant is used to prevent intestinal or respiratory flu and to speed the recovery process along.

In the old days, diseases that caused the body to waste away were called wasting syndromes. The ancients knew which plants would reverse this process and allow the body to build itself back up again, and the jujube was one of these plants. Its fruits are said to increase the flesh and strength of the seriously ill, reversing the process of disease. To my mind, preventative medicine is where it's at, and if the plant can restore a wasting body, one can only imagine what it could do for a reasonably healthy body under stress. The Chinese do stipulate, however, that the jujube should only be used fresh in wasting conditions, as it can cause fever otherwise.

In modern Chinese medicine, the jujube is used to tone the spleen and stomach, to treat shortness of breath and severe emotional upset and debility due to nerves, and to mask the flavors of unpleasant-tasting herbs. Scientists have found that mice fed jujube gained more weight and did markedly better in endurance tests than those not given the fruit. When rabbits exposed to carbon tetrachloride consumed jujube teas daily for a week, they recovered faster than a control group. Also indicative of jujube's positive effect on the liver was a test in which rabbits fed a toxic chemical recovered much more rapidly after consuming jujube than those that did not eat the fruit. What's more, jujube improved the liver function of patients suffering from hepatitis and cirrhosis.

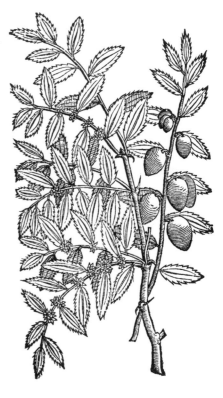

Jujube pits, when aged for three years, are considered excellent for wounds and abdominal pain. The leaves are used to treat children suffering from typhoid fever—they induce the sweating thought to break the fever. They are also used for a number of infectious diseases. The heartwood is considered a powerful blood tonic. The root is used to promote hair growth and in treating such eruptive fevers of children as smallpox, measles, and chicken pox. Last but not least, the bark is used to make an eye wash for inflamed eyes. We might as well call this one the medicine tree.

Although we Westerners have largely forgotten all about the jujube, its medicinal worth was recognized enough in Europe at one time that it received a mention from Gerard in the 17th century. He seems to have felt the same way the Asians do about jujube—it's an excellent tonic for all the parts that matter, especially the lungs and the kidneys:

The fruit of the jujube tree eaten is of hard digestion, and nourisheth very little; but being taken in syrups, electuaries, and such like confections, it appealeth and smootheth the roughness of the throat, the breast and lungs, and is good against the cough, but exceeding good for the reines of the back, and kidneys and bladder.

The Indians and Pakistanis agree that jujube is a fine blood cleanser and a great addition to any diet, particularly if one is prone to illness. Both cultures use the plant as an overall tonic, strengthener, and disease preventer.

Did you ever notice that when you get run down, you get sick, and sometimes once you get sick, you keep getting sick? First it's a sinus infection, then it's an ear infection, then it's a chest cold, and then you get the flu. Have you ever been sick off and on again for a whole season? This seems to be more and more common, and it's just the phenomenon for which the Indians and Pakistanis use jujubes.

JUJUBE. Like the date, the jujube can be eaten out of hand, and this is perhaps the best way to sample its deliciousness as well as its health benefits—buy a bag of jujubes and eat them. They also can be cooked down into a jam if you like to spread your fruit. Just substitute dried jujubes in a recipe for strawberry jam. Before you start the recipe, the jujubes will have to be peeled and stewed. Cut out their olivelike pits, and add one half a cup of water to each cup of jujubes. Then place them over low heat until the fruit has hydrated.

They definitely belong in our tonic. Jujubes are readily available at Asian grocery stores and pharmacies, and if you don't have one in your city or town, there are mail-order Chinese herbal supply companies that will send you as many jujubes as you could ever use. Don't try to substitute the over-the-movie-refreshment-counter variety. It won't work.

Better than buying your jujubes, you might as well grow your own. Any one of several varieties of jujube trees can be had by picking up the phone and calling a mail-order nursery. The shapely tree is a great addition to the yard. With the look of a Japanese weeping cherry tree, it is as decorative as its fruit is edible. In addition, the tree produces bumper crops of fruit and never has to be sprayed for anything. That's right, a fruiting tree that is not subject to the ravages of a million insects. Squirrels, known as tree rats to some, do like the fruit, but it is produced in such quantities that there is enough for everybody.

One of the problems with most fruit trees is that they produce a million pounds of fruit in a week-long period, which means you have to process a lot of fruit all in one day. Not so the jujube. Jujubes will dry right on the tree so that by the time the fruit falls off, you can pop it in a jar for later use.

▼▼▼▼▼▼▼▼▼▼▼▼▼▼▼▼▼▼▼▼▼▼▼

JUNIPER
Juniperus communis

The story of juniper is filled with history. In Europe 200 years ago, juniper was thought to be extremely strengthening to the body: it was administered to the sick to restore, and to the well to maintain good health.

Juniper's most common usage was in a liqueur called junivere, made from juniper berries. People found that when the berries were collected and floated in alcohol, the health agent in the berries was transferred to the liquid, which is more readily consumed than the berries. They're actually more like pine cones (the juniper is a relation of the pine tree) than what we usually associate with the word "berry." Their flavor is quite similar to that of a pine cone, and about as palatable—you don't just pick them off the tree and have a good chew.

The best junivere was said to be made by the Dutch. The liqueur was one of the most popular tonics in Europe at the time Europeans began colonizing the world, and as they traveled the globe, it came with them. As nasty as it was for the white man to move into other people's countries and take over for financial exploitation, the native diseases they encountered there were almost as bad, and administered a little justice. Death rates were phenomenal, folks became extremely health- or, more importantly, staying-well-conscious, and junivere was but one of the many tonics or restoratives which became popular in the colonies.

The gin and tonic dates to this era. As the British plundered India, they fell subject to malaria. The preventative medicine of the day was a combination of juniper berries in the form of gin, the British equivalent of the Dutch junivere, and water flavored with quinine, the leading anti-malarial agent. Though the beverage has become a country club favorite, its roots are purely medicinal. The various Bombay gins sold now trace their origins back to India and the time when juniper and tonic water were taken on a daily basis to avoid coming down with malaria.

Today, the berries used as the flavoring agent in gin come from the European juniper bush, *Juniperus communis*, but the juniper family has a number of relations worldwide, and many of these have been recognized for their power to heal. The ancient Israelites are said to have known the juniper, as it grows in the mountains all over the Near East, and the Arabs of today use the oil of the plant to treat liver afflictions and as a general tonic.

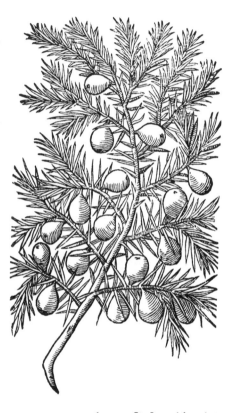

The people of India were already quite familiar with the plant long before the British arrived; they believe the berries to be tonic, stimulating, and especially good for the kidneys. They also toss them into the curry pot for health and flavor.

In North America, the Micmac and Malecite Indians, native to the maritime provinces of Canada, used *Juniperus communis* for sprains, wounds, tuberculosis, ulcers both internal and external, consumption, and rheumatism. Their general belief was that the juniper hardened the body and made it better at fighting off illness. Less universally accepted, but perhaps more intriguing is the use to which juniper berries are put by practitioners of hoodoo in the Louisiana bayou. St. Joseph's mixture, which also includes buds from the garden of Gilead (poplar buds), berries of fish (bayberries), wishing beans (tonka beans), Japanese scented lucky beans (jequirity beans), and star anise, features the pineconelike fruits. Of course, as witch doctors tend to be cagey people, it's hard to track down the exact purpose of the ointment and the nature of its various ingredients, but all of them are aromatic, and the potion is used in conjuring—a before-magic bath splash, if you will.

In South America, a different juniper is used for various conditions and as a general tonic. The notion of making booze with juniper berries is obviously a popular one—the South Americans brew up a cocktail called *ade*, which they take for staying well. Whereas the European gin is merely flavored with juniper berries, the South American version is actually fermented from juniper berries mixed with sugar and, in some countries, aloe vera. The berries are also made into jams and marmalades, an objectionable notion if you ask me. Imagine a blob of sweetened pine cones smeared on your breakfast toast. To each his own.

In case you should ever find yourself in a situation where you are being attacked by parasitic catfish, juniper may help you out. It seems that the Cuna Indians have a fretful time with a variety of fish that swim up and attach themselves to the genitals to suck blood. When you're out for a bath, this can mean the end of the party, and so the Cuna smear themselves with the berries to repel the nasty varmints. Between piranhas, these catfish, and boa constrictors, I think on my next trip to South America I'll stick to the hotel pool.

The South Americans, along with the rest of the world, use ground berries and other parts of the juniper as what is essentially a local antibiotic to treat wounds and sores. There is some scientific basis to this as the phenol contained in the plant is actually a bacteria killer which would indeed keep a wound safe from infection.

Despite the fact that eating juniper berries is like chewing pine-flavored gum, they have been used for food at various points in history. The Native Americans preferred the California juniper (*Juniperus californica*), the Utah juniper (*Juniperus utahensis*), and the check-barked or alligator juniper (*Juniperus pachyphlaea*). When I say food, I should add that the berries were not eaten the way we eat strawberries. Instead, they were dried, ground into a pine-scented meal, then shaped into patties, and fried. This gets the bonus yuck rating in my book. Apparently, though, the cakes would keep body and soul together, they were easy to digest, and the Native Americans found that these juniper fritters stimulated the flow of urine in a big way.

JUNIPER. This is another truly medicinal plant, with little or no redeeming flavor features. I don't drink alcohol, so gin and tonics are out of the question for me. However, I do use an old European recipe for a nonalcoholic juniper syrup which, when added to tonic water, tastes almost the same as a gin and tonic. Boil one cup of berries with one gallon of water for half an hour, strain the berries out, add four cups of sugar, and boil the liquid again for five minutes. Store the syrup in the refrigerator. When I'm feeling run down, I pour myself a "gin and tonic," sit out on the porch, and relax.

Apart from its use as a food and a tonic, the Native Americans used juniper for gynecological health. The Zunis made a tea from the toasted branches to relax a woman's muscles before child-birth began and to speed her recovery from the delivery. The Tewa Indians burned the branches in the dwelling of a woman who had just given birth. The Spanish Americans, who learned of the native plant from various indigenous tribes, advised that women drink a cup or so of the tea a month before their babies were due to assure a safe delivery. In addition, the same Southwesterners used the tea to treat an inflamed stomach and relieve muscle spasms.

Not to get personal or anything, but did you ever notice that a good gin and tonic sends you to the rest room more than usual? I know that bathroom talk is a no-no in Western society since none of us do that. However, in the interest of science, I raise the topic. Juniper is, in fact, a fairly powerful diuretic. The berries and the liquors flavored with them flush out the kidneys, which is generally a good thing to have happen in our toxic-ridden world. Some herbalists feel that juniper berries will further irritate existing kidney problems, so if you have kidney troubles, you may want to avoid this one.

Speaking of tidying up our interiors, juniper also acts as an intestinal antiseptic. As Europeans colonized the world, they came into contact with what we now call Montezuma's Revenge. The root cause of this condition, unpleasant enough with modern facilities and a nightmare in more rustic days, is having unfamiliar beasts take up residence in the intestinal tract. The colonists were right on when they drank gin every day, as were the Spanish Americans who drank juniper tea for stomach spasms—it would have indeed killed anything down the pipes that had no business being there.

Modern gin is relatively low in juniper content—the extract is usually somewhere around .01 percent and the juniper oil content somewhere around .006 percent. If you want to make a beverage that is higher in juniper content, and thus in medicinal power, float a cup of juniper berries in some commercial gin for a few months. Still and all, alcohol is hell on the liver, and despite the fact that the old-time healers preferred their juniper with "fire water," there are healthier ways to take it.

For our tonic, we will be using juniper berries, fresh or dried. They're easy to come by—pick some up at the grocery store spice shelf, or plant a juniper tree for a ready source. As with all our ingredients, the fresher, the better, and what could be fresher than berries from your own tree? Run to the garden center and ask for a *Juniperus communis* tree, plant according to instructions, and within a year or two, go out with your bowl and pick away.

LEMON BALM

Melissa officinalis

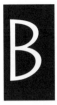eing overwrought is a bad thing anyhow you cut it. The modern world works our nerves to the edge, and that's when our bodies give into disease, be it a cold or worse. Being uptight all the time is said to cause all sorts of ills, from heart disease and cancer to stomach disorders and allergies. To repeat myself, stress kills. Slowing down and chilling out could save your life.

People need to relax, and their bodies need it too. Unfortunately, many choose to do so under the influence of alcohol, street drugs, and the tranquilizers Western doctors pass out like vitamins. These substances are as bad for the body as the original condition of tension. Our next plant, lemon balm, could help you out on this front. What's more, it's nonaddicting and won't corrode your liver or your brain.

This plant soothes the body without ravaging it at the same time. *Balm.* Even the word is soothing. Like lip, lemon balm is a comforting substance. It smoothes the mind rather than the lips, but the concept is the same. Since antiquity, lemon balm has been used in healing, particularly in healing the mind, which controls everything.

Have you ever encountered a mintlike plant that emits a lemony smell when you crush it? That's lemon balm. The plant has been around so long that no one is quite clear where it started out, but today it grows all over the world, partly due to its reputation as a panacea, partly due to its vigorous growth.

A relation of the mint, lemon balm is perhaps one of the most widely used herbs outside of the United States. A hundred years ago, Americans used it medicinally too. A classic blood purifier was made out of lemon balm, yarrow, saffron, and mountain rush. The ingredients were boiled together for a tea said to clean the body of impurities and restore health. Today, we don't do this anymore, and Americans treat lemon balm like it's another weed.

In looking backward to discover forgotten information, a traditional concept we see over and over again is that illnesses are caused by impurities in the body and that if the body can be cleansed, health will return. Though we tend to dismiss the old health ways as ridiculous, we are starting to learn scientifically that this idea is not far from the truth. Exposure to and absorption of toxic materials, whether chemical or viral, cause illness.

Though we have confirmed what everybody knew 100 years ago about internal body cleansing, we are only starting to learn what they also knew about which plants would do the tidying. Lemon balm was one of these plants.

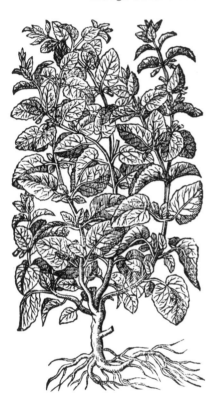

Contrary to popular belief, lemon balm is not the plant referred to in the Bible as the Balm of Gilead. The biblical balm comes from the sticky buds of a Near Eastern poplar tree. The ancient Israelites apparently didn't know about lemon balm, and that's a pity. However, the Arabs of today are quite familiar with it. They make it into a delightful tea which they serve sweet and find to be an antiviral, antispasmodic, and stomach toning agent. The most interesting property is its antiviral action, but hold on to your seats, we will get to that later.

The Spanish are quite fond of lemon balm. Like people around the world, they feel that it is a calming plant. Today we believe that a big part of staying healthy is being kind and gentle to one's self. The Spanish second the motion and recommend boiling a pot of lemon balm, adding the juice to a hot bath, and sitting in the warm water to rest the body and mind. When they moved into South America, they brought lemon balm along with them. The Venezuelans feel that the plant aids in digestion and helps overweight people shed a few pounds. The plant is also applied to any skin problems, including wounds, sores, and skin ulcers.

Like their Spanish ancestors, South Americans use lemon balm to treat a wide variety of nervous complaints and symptoms of stress. They feel that balm tea or, better yet, balm tea drunk during a balm bath defines soothing. Whenever tension enters the scene, South Americans reach for lemon balm the way North

Thirty Plants That Can Save Your Life!

Americans reach for aspirin, one important difference being that lemon balm won't burn the stomach and aspirin will.

Now let's get to some scientific facts. Newcastle disease, mumps, herpes simplex, and vaccinia have all suffered at the hands of lemon balm. The polyphenols contained in the plant are said to be the active ingredients in this process, but who really cares what little chemical does the trick? The fact is that the plant is antiviral, and most viruses cause downtime.

The plant has also proven to be antibacterial along with having antihistaminic and antispasmodic properties. The antibacterial effect is quite interesting in that one of the oldest uses for lemon balm is as a paste to prevent the infection of wounds. Along these lines, Gerard had a few choice words:

Smiths Bawme or Carpenters Bawme is most singular to heal up green wounds that are cut with iron; it cureth the rupture in short time; it stayeth the whites. Dioscorides and Pliny have attributed like virtues unto this kind of bawme, which they call iron wort. The leaves (say they) being applied, close up wounds without any peril of inflammation. Pliny saith that it is of so great virtue that though it be but tied to his sword that hath given the wound, it stancheth the blood.

LEMON BALM. Unlike some of our other tonic plants, lemon balm is a pleasure to drink. My favorite use for it is in what I call the "Lemon Special." Add four cups of lemon balm leaves to one quart of boiling water and turn the heat off. Save one cup to drink and dump the rest in a tub filled with hot water. Sip the tea while resting in the lemon-fresh bath. This is an old beauty treatment that has fallen out of use in recent years, but I think it's high time for a revival.

Gerard also praised lemon balm as a mental-health plant, asserting that, "Bawme drunke in wine is good against the bitings of venomous beasts, comforts the heart, and driveth away all melancholy and sadness." To think that our lawn-care companies have developed a special herbicide just to kill lemon balm is shocking!

The Shakers, who were quite fond of lemon balm, grew and sold it in great quantities in the mid-1800s. The plant has both a lemony scent and a distinctly lemony flavor, and when crushed in water and sweetened, it makes a very relaxing summertime drink. If lemons weren't so good for you, I would suggest that we trade in traditional lemonade for the kind made with lemon balm, which, it could be argued, is even better for the body. Apparently, the Quakers like to take rest breaks from the summer's heat with a cooling toddy of lemon balm and honey.

Another use for the plant is in female reproductive health. Lemon balm is said to be a real boon to women, making menstruating, giving birth, and even conceiving much easier. In New Zealand, lemon balm is considered to be mother's little helper in every sense of the word—any problem with the secret parts, as Gerard would say, is helped out with lemon balm. While we are down there, lemon balm is also considered excellent for bladder problems, which we all know are bad things to have.

It's sad that such a soothing, beneficial herb is now on the most-wanted list at garden centers coast to coast, but the truth is that lemon balm is one invasive plant. You don't grow lemon balm, you control it. I once had two herb beds separated by a slab of concrete, which was parted in two by a seam put in when the concrete was laid some 30 years earlier. The lemon balm spread from one herb bed to the other via this crack, popping up where a piece of concrete was missing.

With lemon balm, a little in the garden goes a long way, although using it will certainly help keep it under control. You can purchase lemon balm at the garden center, or take a start from a friend's garden regardless of the season. The good news is that one start planted in the garden will soon produce more than enough herb to take care of your tension headaches all year round.

▼▼▼▼▼▼▼▼▼▼▼▼▼▼▼▼▼▼▼▼▼▼▼

LICORICE
Glycyrrhiza glabra

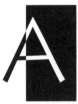s I've said before, the top medicinal plants are special in various ways, if not downright bizarre. They tend to have some obvious peculiarity, something so strange that it's easy to know how people were initially drawn to them. Take licorice, for example. The root contains glycorisin, a substance 50 times sweeter than sugar. How's that for an odd fact? When you put a piece of licorice in your mouth and experience the ultra-sweet taste, you know that something is up with this plant.

Are we talking about licorice sticks? Yes, but not the ones you buy at the five-and-dime. Not so long ago, a few hundred years or thereabout, sugar as we know it did not exist. It was not that people didn't have a sweet tooth: the white stuff was not available. Before the days of colonialism and the cane sugar plantation, folks had to rely on fruit, honey, or licorice sticks—the real variety. These sticks come from the roots of a member of the bean family, and people used to chew on them for their flavor, which is truly sickeningly sweet.

Far beyond being a treat, however, licorice was, and in some countries still is, used to bring on health and a robust appearance, so much so that too much can cause weight gain. If you are trying to lose a few pounds, licorice is not the plant for you. Conversely, if you want to put on a few, it is what you've been looking for.

Licorice is nothing new. In fact, it was mentioned by Oribasius and Marcellus in the fourth century, A.D., and by Paul of Aegina in the seventh. By the time the 15th century rolled around, Italy was famous for its superior licorice—in 1574, Mattioli noted that pastilles flavored with its juice were brought every year from Apulia. Indeed, the record of this substance indicates that it has been an article of domestic and medicinal use for centuries. According to some historians, licorice was stored in King Tut's tomb. (Remember, the pharaohs only traveled to the next life with the best and most necessary stuff.)

In the Arab world, the consensus is: whatever ails you, use licorice. The extensive list of indications includes fever, respiratory ailments, and gastritis. One Arab use is to take licorice root, carob pulp, and raisins, grind them all together, and freeze them into a healthful sherbet. As the other two ingredients, carob and raisins, are also powerful health plants, the combination is a winner.

In China, licorice is felt to boost the body, any body: long-term usage leads to clear eyes and vibrancy. The Chinese believe that the herb enters through the lung and spleen channels, and as such is specifically good for both. They see licorice as a herbal helper, if you will, and they use it in most of their prescriptions to add power to the other herbs they contain. For example, if you are taking angelica for female complaints, the addition of licorice will make the angelica all the more effective. In Chinese medicine, as we have discussed, health is defined as the body in balance. Herbs are used to bring balance back, and licorice is considered the balancer of herbs. It's termed a corrective, a fancy word which means that the plant corrects what's wrong with you, whatever that may be.

The claims of licorice being a universal healer or panacea are so numerous that the scientific community has spent a considerable piece of lab time trying to figure out what in the plant makes it so good for the body. The list of chemicals they've isolated in the sweet root goes on and on. I will spare you the details, but researchers have verified many of the so-called old wives' tales surrounding the plant. Their scrutiny has backed up what the villagers already knew.

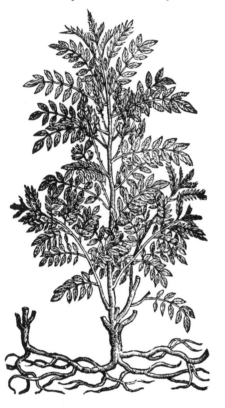

Being a man and never having had to deal with a monthly period, I cannot even imagine what a bother erratic menstruation can be. A traditional treatment for irregular cycling, licorice has been proven to induce the production of estrogen, the hormone that regulates estrus.

We all know that a stomachache can be debilitating—it's hard to sit in an important meeting when all you want to do is lie down and die. At the risk of sounding like an idiot, I'll say that the stomach is a really important organ. Without nourishment, we starve to death, and the stomach is the instrument that introduces nutrition into the body. I bother making such a remedial statement because the way many people treat their stomachs suggests that they're not in touch with this fact. Be good to your stomach, and your body will be good to you. Licorice is considered one of the best plants for the overall health of the stomach and is used universally to treat stomach ulcers.

Chinese scientists have proven that licorice extract actually does cure ulcers, and it does so through two means. First, it absorbs the acid content in the stomach, making it much more ph-balanced, and second, it relaxes the stomach and intestines, thus relieving spasms. They have found licorice to be, are you ready, 90 percent effective in the treatment of ulcers. Apparently the best course of action is to take the powdered root at the onset of an attack, rather than waiting until it is full-blown. Sounds like preventative medicine to me, and ulcer sufferers might be wise to follow this Chinese advice.

A folk cure for cancer in a number of cultures, licorice has been proven to inhibit the growth of sarcoma 45 and Ehrlich ascites cells. Aside from its ability to inhibit actual cancer cell growth, the plant is used to boost the body so that it can fight off degenerative conditions, of which cancer is certainly one. In the case of debilitating diseases, it has been shown that licorice administered in the early phases of the disease leads to weight gain and improvement of strength, blood pressure, and general well being. The key here again is to take licorice early, as a preventative, to avoid going all the way down the tubes.

The notion that licorice fights inflammatory conditions due to arthritis or rheumatism is universally held. As it turns out, the plant contains a number of chemicals which have proven to be anti-inflammatory in lab animals. Scientists are now making a connection between inflammatory diseases and allergic reactions, and in Asia licorice is used to treat allergies with great success. The active ingredients in licorice have been shown to decrease allergic reactions in guinea pigs. For the inflammatory disease sufferer who also has allergies, the plant is considered supreme.

In *Macer Floridus*, a ninth-century herbalist declares, "No medecyne helpith swether pe instrumentis of pe lunges, ne of pe brest, pan dop liquorice." More succinctly put, no plant is better for the lungs than licorice. Science has born this out. An ingredient in licorice is said to be comparable to codeine for coughs. At one time, singers used to chew the root to strengthen the throat and protect their sources of income, and asthmatics took the same plant to help them breathe. A modern study shows that the symptoms of patients suffering from bronchial asthma were relieved within three days after the administration of powdered licorice.

LICORICE. This is—how shall I put it—an acquired taste. The first bite can be brutally sweet. I chew licorice root straight from the package as soon as I get that achy feeling which means a cold is about to set in. By chewing (I mean swallowing the juice until all the sweetness is gone and then spitting out the pulp) one stick an hour and getting a good night's sleep, I find that I can usually avoid a full-blown cold. Even though I can only handle a bit at a time, you can chew as much licorice as you like, but keep in mind that it has been known to make gaining weight easier.

When researchers noted all the references to the plant's power to cure infectious diseases, they started looking for antibiotic properties in the licorice stick, and—surprise, surprise—they discovered an ingredient called triterpenoid glycyrrhetic acid which indeed kills bacteria. Another chemical, hispaglabridin, was also found to be potent against bacteria. We've all seen these cold formulas advertised on TV with seven million and one different actions: cough suppressant, decongestant, etc. Well, licorice is a cold formula made by Mother Nature herself which has all of the above, plus an antibiotic.

Licorice sticks, the real kind, can be purchased from your local herb seller or readily grown. Incredibly hardy, the plant is an attractive shrub which rarely gets larger than an azalea bush. One-year-old plants are easily available from mail-order sources. Remember, though, that the part to use is the root, and if you are planting for roots, you need to make sure you can readily get them out of the ground as they can be as long as 16 feet. The best course is to prepare a special bed by mixing a huge bag of peat moss in with the garden soil so that the soil is light and fluffy. Then, when it's time to harvest, you can actually pull the roots out with no trouble. After you trim off the roots, stick the plant back into the ground, and it will grow anew.

▼▼▼▼▼▼▼▼▼▼▼▼▼▼▼▼▼▼▼▼▼▼▼

MINT
Mentha piperita

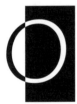n a trip to the Middle East, I had the chance to travel with some Bedouin traders. As my friends stopped in different villages to do business, I first became acquainted with mint tea. At each stop, the woman of the house would disappear into the kitchen and return with glass cups of the hot drink. On another trip to northern Spain, I was interested to note that every restaurant offered mint tea, or *poleo* as it is called, as an after-dinner beverage along with coffee.

Even in the United States, a bowl of mints can be seen at almost every restaurant cash register. Take a look at the candy rack at your local convenience store, and you will find an overabundance of mint products. Mint is everywhere and used by everyone. Did you ever wonder why or how this after-dinner-mint thing got started? Well, go ahead and ask yourself the question, and I will be so kind as to answer it for you. The fact is that we are surrounded by mint for a very good reason: it's one of the most widely used tonics in the world.

Mint is the stomach tonic plant. It helps the stomach to feel better and work better too. Did you ever wonder where the idea for mint jelly came from? Currently we see it in bright green blobs served with lamb, but formerly its use was more widespread. The tradition dates back to the orgiastic feasts of medieval Europe where whole pigs and cows were served along with birds innumerable. A day of gorging on heavy meats was apt to give all included a bellyache, but folks discovered that if the meats were eaten with jellies spirited with mint, stomachaches were eliminated or at least reduced. Subsequent research has shown that the oils in mint help to break down fats and make them more readily digested. Open any herbal, and you will see the same comment about mint, that it "aids in digestion." As digestion is the core of living, anything that helps us digest our food is something we need to look into.

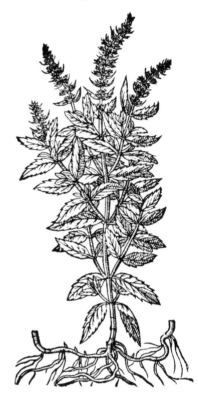

The word *mint* is a general term for a group of closely related plants that all have one thing in common: when bruised or scratched, they emit the characteristic mint smell. There are more mints than a person could shake a stick at—peppermint, spearmint, Egyptian mint, mint of cologne, anise mint, Japanese mint, watermint—the list goes on. The two most widely grown mints are peppermint and spearmint, but regardless of type, all mints have the desired effect on the stomach: good health.

Mint is an old plant, so old that no one really knows when it was first used, but it doesn't take a rocket scientist to figure out how the ancients first noticed the aromatic herb. Mint was used as medicine in England as early as the ninth century. A book said to have been written some time around 849 A.D. asserts not only that mint comforts the stomach, but also that it kills worms, cures earaches, heals skin ulcers, dog bites, and head wounds, and increases the milk in lactating mothers. What's more, European sources insist that it assures the conception of male children when consumed and acts as a contraception when placed in the vagina. Who would have guessed?

In Latin America, mint is known as *yerbabuena*, or the good herb. The New World Latins developed a taste for mint from their Spanish ancestors who brought the plant over from the Old World; they see mint as a supreme tonic to use in the case of illnesses that won't go away and, of course, to avoid getting sick in the first place. In these parts, whatever ails you gets treated first with mint tea: difficult labor, miscarriage, menstrual cramps, colic, stomachache, diarrhea, kidney and urinary tract infections, toothache, earache, poison ivy, pimples, rashes, colds, fevers, and fright. As I said, mint is used for just about everything.

In Djakarta, mint grows wild all over the place and is used for two things, headaches and colds. The leaves are ground with a bit of lime and poulticed on the temples for relief from a throbbing head. The same leaves are brewed for a serious cough, and when a person takes the chills, mint is used immediately. In New Zealand, mint is used as a tonic and to treat colds, flu, headaches, colic, gas, and nausea. Oil of peppermint put on burns quickly relieves the pain, and taken on a regular basis, it is said to dissolve gallstones.

MINT. While I was traveling in the Arab states, I developed a taste for sweetened mint tea with bread for an afternoon snack. My recipe for the tea is to gather mint fresh from the garden, dump it into a pot of boiling water, and allow it to simmer for five or ten minutes. Use one cup of fresh mint leaves for every three cups of water (if it's dried, use one teaspoon per cup). The Arabs add three or four teaspoons of sugar to each cup of tea; I prefer one tablespoon of honey.

In China, *Mentha arvensis* or *po-ho* is the local mint used in healing as it has been for at least a thousand years. With it, the Chinese treat fevers, flu, colds, nosebleeds, diseases of the nose and throat, snake and insect bites, and nervous disorders of children. There, as in many parts of Asia, mint is used as a salad green and added to vegetable dishes. The Vietnamese use fresh mint along with watercress as an appetizer served early in the meal so that the mint will get the stomach functioning and ready for the onslaught of food.

The Indians use *Mentha arvensis* to tone the stomach, stimulate the mind and body, rid the intestines of unsocial gas, and relieve muscular spasms. Yet another nation sees the plant as being the original friend of the stomach, and they crush it to add to fruit chutneys. In India, chutney is more than a condiment, it is a tonic taken with each meal to ensure good health. What other herbs go into chutney? Oh, garlic, mustard, ginger, cinnamon, to name a few. Do these sound familiar? Rather than take tonic formulas, the Indians eat their tonics right along with dinner. Believe it or not, our mustard and ketchup descend from the same practice.

The Arabs use *Mentha spicata*, *Mentha villosa*, and *Mentha suaveole* for many ailments, including diseases of the skin. They see mint as the supreme refresher of the body, and they should know: they deal with hot, dry weather on a daily basis. The cups of mint tea I drank on my trip to the Bedouin camps were served for this reason—mint peps up weary travelers. Halfway across the globe, the Mennonites also beat the heat with big pitchers of mint tea. The Southerners seem to prefer mint juleps, with a little whiskey added to make the drink more annihilating, but the basic idea is the same: to keep you cool when the temperature isn't.

A friend of mine trapped in the legal profession recently told me he needed a mental mint. He meant that his life seemed stale and needed some refreshment, but unbeknownst to him, mint may have been precisely what his situation called for. The Arabs are only one of many peoples who feel mint is a mind as well as a stomach tonic. Mint is one tea that can jump-start the mind into a more energetic state, minus the shakes that many of our stimulating beverages offer.

For the sake of our stomachs, mint will be included in our tonic mixture, as well as for the sake of our taste buds. Some of the ingredients are pretty nasty tasting, and mint is a great cover-up. As to getting the mint for our use, there is no excuse for not growing the plant yourself. But wait, that statement is not even true. There is no excuse for not putting some mint in the garden and letting it grow itself. This is a weed plant along the lines of burdock and dandelion, and a fresh supply couldn't be easier to have—just get a start from a friend and stick it in the ground. For tonic-making purposes, the plant can be picked and tossed in the pot whenever it is green. This is, by the way, most of the year.

▼▼▼▼▼▼▼▼▼▼▼▼▼▼▼▼▼▼▼▼▼▼▼

MUSTARD
Brassica nigra

hen you see the word *mustard*, what usually comes to mind is the yellow stuff that gets plastered on a bun before the hot dog. This is the very substance that could save your life.

There are several different types of this health-giving plant: white mustard, black mustard, and leaf mustard. The white and the black are raised for their seeds, and the leaf, as one might guess, is raised for its tender greens. The yellow stuff that comes in bottles with squeeze holes is the ground seed of black mustard, usually mixed with vinegar and a host of secret ingredients. The idea of mustard seed paste is universal, but each and every culture adds its own touch to the mixture. The common ingredient is mustard flour or sinapine; the materials that keep the mustard glued together are what vary from country to

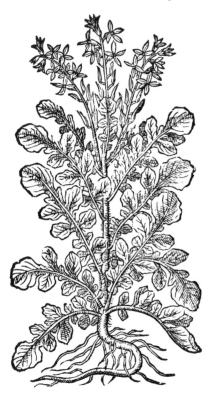

country. The French make their mustard with whole berries and white wine vinegar, the Chinese make theirs with rice wine vinegar, and the Americans make theirs with artificial flavorings, preservatives, and yellow dye. By the way, mustard is not naturally yellow, and mustard that is bright yellow is colored with something that probably isn't a tonic by nature.

The mustard plant is a relation of cabbage and broccoli, a member of the family that's gotten so much press lately as being anticancer. The condiment mustard has its roots in health, and all of the cultures that smear it on their sandwiches originally did so to preserve their well-being. The paste was thought to aid in digestion and lead to extra vitality.

Hey, next time you have the mustard out for a sandwich, take your shoes and socks off and smear some on the bottoms of your feet— it's an old European country cure for bodily debility. Who knows, it may work. Mustard plasters are an official treatment to reduce fever worldwide. I must say that I would never have thought to use mustard on anything other than corned beef, but scratch the surface in the mustard arena, and you will be surprised what you find.

White mustard (*Sinapis alba*) seems to be indigenous to the southern countries of Europe and Western Asia, from which, according to Chinese authors, it was introduced into China. Formerly it was not distinguished from black mustard. Like black mustard, over which it is preferred on account of its color and mildness, white mustard is an exceedingly popular stimulating condiment.

Black mustard (*Brassica nigra*) is found over the whole of Europe, excepting

Thirty Plants That Can Save Your Life!

the extreme north. It also abounds in northern Africa, Asia Minor, the Caucasian region, western India, southern Siberia, and China, as well as in North and South America, where it is now naturalized. Known to the ancients, it seems to have been used more as a medicine than as a condiment in early times, but in 300 B.C., Diocletian spoke of its use with food in the eastern part of the Roman Empire. During the Middle Ages, Europeans esteemed it as an accompaniment to salted meats. They found that mustard, like mint, aided the digestion. Gerard was talking about eating it with meats in 1696, as we do to this day.

Leaf mustard has been developed for use as a salad and cooking green. It is more widely used in Asia than in the United States, but anyone with a relative in the South has been offered a plate of the mushy stuff alongside fried chicken.

The familiar saying, enough is enough, is quite appropriate in the case of mustard: a little mustard guarantees health, a little too much mustard, and you can plan to spend the day hanging over the john, losing what health you once had. You see, mustard has been used both as a tonic and as a purging agent. The rule of thumb is that if you've taken too much, your stomach will most kindly fill you in.

Like vomiting, constipation is an ugly experience, and in the Tennessee hills where, as in other rural parts of the United States, wild mustard is a traditional spring tonic herb, every mother has a number of tricks up her sleeve to speed the elimination process along. One recipe uses one tablespoon of ground white mustard seed mixed with a syrup made of four cups of water and two cups of honey, to be taken a tablespoon at a time, once a day. The Arabs use a similar concoction for the same problem.

In 1475, Bjornsson had this to say about our favorite relish: "mustard whets a man's wits, and it loosens the belly, breaks the stones, and purges the urine, if one eats mustard, that strengthens the stomach and lessens its sickness. Crushed mustard in vinegar heals vipers bite. With mustard one may cauterize." Along these lines, mustard is widely used in South America to induce vigor. The leaves are laid on skin afflictions, and the seeds are seen as speedy treatments for liver and spleen complaints. As the plant is packed with volatile

MUSTARD. Making homemade mustard is well worth the effort. Buy a pound of whole mustard seeds from the health-food store and grind half of them in a food processor to a flourlike consistency. Place the other half in a saucepan, add enough white wine vinegar to cover them, and simmer the seeds until tender. Combine the ground mustard with the simmered seeds, adding more white wine vinegar if the mixture is too thick. I always let the mustard age in jars for a few weeks before using it because the longer it rests, the better it gets.

oils with proven antimicrobial properties, both practices make scientific sense.

One of the oldest widespread uses for mustard is in the treatment of colds. As Gerard noted, "It is given with good success in like manner to such as be short winded, and are stopped in the breast with tough flegme from the head and brain." In the southern United States, mustard still factors into home cures for head colds. One informant tells that mustard leaves scalded and applied to the chest will prevent pneumonia, another suggests plasters made of ground mustard seed, and a third recommends a hot foot bath seasoned with ground seed for colds and grippe. A folk cold cure from Utah includes three parts mustard, two parts cornstarch and water. The grandmother who laid this one on us insisted that if you drink this concoction, it will absolutely cure you. It might make you spit up, but it will cure you of your cold just the same.

Aside from colds, mustard has been considered the plant par excellence in treating a bad dose of the rheumatiz, otherwise known as the achy bones and general fatigue sometimes associated with age but not necessarily. Either the mustard is mixed with mutton fat and applied to the affected part, the plant is boiled and the feet are soaked in the resulting warm liquid, or teaspoons of the ground powder are mixed with honey and taken internally. These are also considered effective treatments for paralysis.

This business of using mustard in foot baths is again found in India. The Indians reiterate that mustard is good for fevers and rheumatism, but they also go on to say that it is excellent for general fatigue. The next time you get yourself all worked into a frenzy and feel that special kind of tired that comes on before a cold sets in, fill the spaghetti pan with hot water and freshly ground mustard, and stick in your feet for a spell. The Indians go on to suggest that some mustard be put in the navel at the same time for a double whammy treatment to be done before bed. Once again, it's preventative medicine. I don't know about the navel, but the foot procedure seems worth a try.

One of my favorite uses of mustard also comes from Gerard. "It helpeth those that have their hair pulled off; it taketh away the blue and black marks that come of bruisings." When I read this, I instantly imagine Middle English lads and maidens at the town square, pulling each other's hair out in big clumps and laughing wildly. In case anyone ever pulls your hair out, it's nice to know to get the bottle out and smear some mustard on your head.

On a more serious note, Gerard wraps up the mustard topic with this statement: "The seed of Thlafpi or treacle mustard eaten, purgeth colour both upward and downward." In other words, mustard brings healthy color to the body. This thought is consistent worldwide. Good coloration indicates a healthy body, and that is what mustard can help you achieve.

MYRRH

Commiphora myrrha

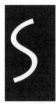everal hundred years ago, some wise men brought the young Christ Child a heavy load of gifts which included frankincense and myrrh. Today, most of us have heard of myrrh because we've heard the Christmas story, but what is it anyway, and how could it save your life?

At the time of Jesus' birth and before, myrrh was considered a sacred substance associated with godliness. In those days, as now, myrrh was used for two things: religious rites and healing. On the religious side, myrrh was used along with frankincense as a popular incense. Burned in the temples, it exudes a most heavenly scent. Now, in order to understand why myrrh was so popular, you have to focus on a few facts. What with open sewage, people and animals sharing beds (remember where Jesus was born), not to mention the fact that bathing on a regular basis wouldn't come into vogue for centuries, the ancient world smelled really bad. Noxious odors abounded, and perfume was a luxury of the super rich. The only sweet-smelling article common people had contact with was fresh flowers. Burning myrrh masked the nastiness. The fragrance was such a shock in the midst of all the stink that people assumed it had to have links with God.

Myrrh is not actually a plant but rather a plant product, one of the oldest plant products still in active use. The commiphora tree, when slit with a knife, exudes a gummy white substance that hardens quickly in the Near Eastern sun. You may have noticed the clear gelatinous substance that cherry trees secrete when attacked by borers. Myrrh is similar, with the important exception that long ago, and we mean really long ago, man discovered the substance is fragrant and when burned creates an incense that puts those who inhale it into a dreamlike state.

Not long ago I got my hands on some myrrh, and my dinner guests and I decided to try lighting the ancient gum in an incense burner. As it flamed away, putting out its luxurious smoke, a dull quiet spread over the room. Who knows what was so soothing to me and my guests, but the incense definitely made

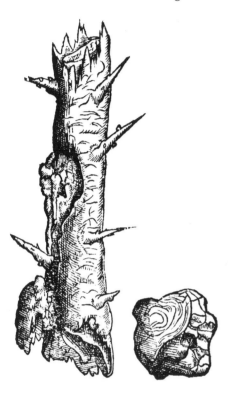

everyone feel like nap time. Ten adults went from chatting noisily to sitting quietly enjoying the silence. Myrrh does something to the human mind. We are only now learning about pheromones, little chemicals that are sucked in by the nose and affect the brain, and after seeing what myrrh did to my dinner party, I am inclined to think that there is something inside the gum which puts the human mind in a special place.

Though the plant is revered by all cultures familiar with it, the myths attached to its creation are less than noble. The leading one holds that Myrrha, daughter of a king of Cyprus, developed an unnatural fixation on her father, a desire that even people in the days of human sacrifice found out of line. We are talking about the big taboo. As she wouldn't let up on her yen for dear old dad, he banished her to the barren deserts of Arabia where the gods transformed her into a myrrh tree exuding tears sweet with repentance.

When I say that myrrh has been kicking around for some time, I mean serious business. In the fifth century, B.C., Herodotus noted that the Egyptians used myrrh in embalming:

First with a crooked iron they draw out the brains through the nostrils, extracting it partly thus and partly by pouring in drugs; and after this with a sharp stone of Ethiopia they make a cut along the side and take out the whole contents of the belly, and when they have cleared out the cavity and cleansed it with palm-wine they cleanse it again with spices pounded up; then they fill the belly with pure

Thirty Plants That Can Save Your Life!

myrrh pounded up and with cassia and other spices except frankincense, and sew it together again.

A more appealing quotation about myrrh comes from the Bible:

I rose up to open up to my beloved, and my hands dropped with myrrh, and my fingers with sweet smelling myrrh, upon the handles of the lock. His cheeks are as a bed of spices, as sweet flowers, his lips like lilies, dropping sweet smelling myrrh.

Sounds like the sound track to a racy sex film? Wrong, Song of Songs, chapter 5: verse 5. Look it up, you will see it plain as day. *Mor*, as the ancient Hebrews called it, receives not one, but eleven biblical listings.

Myrrh is a good example of how when a plant finds use in both religion and healing, they are really one and the same. Myrrh's specialness is hard to tack down and put into words. To understand myrrh, you have to buy some, let it burn in the house, and experience its presence. The Wise Men felt its essential value so strongly that they deemed it a worthy gift for the newborn Christ Child, and they were right.

Medicinally, myrrh has been used as a stimulant, antiseptic, expectorant, antispasmodic, emmenagogue, and stomachic. Conditions for which it is recommended include cancers, leprosy, syphilitic ulcers, sores, sore throats, asthma, coughs, bad breath, weak gums, and loose

MYRRH. After a hectic day, I like to take a jar of myrrh and head to the bathroom. I put one teaspoon in a tub of hot water and a little more in an incense burner. Then I step into the bath and marinate as I take in the ancient incense's fragrance. After about 20 minutes into the procedure, I find that my perspective on life has taken a definite turn for the better. Myrrh does wonders for both the skin and the mind, and soaking it in is a great way to preserve mental health, which is one of the keys to staying well.

teeth. It is currently used mainly in treating such conditions involving bleeding, pain, and wounds as hemorrhoids, menstrual difficulties, tumors, and arthritis. The list goes on.

In China, myrrh is used to correct defective health and as a sedative. Like people in other cultures, the Chinese use it to treat wounds and ulcers. They believe that the herb, which enters the body through the liver channel, invigorates the blood and gets it moving rapidly to all the different body parts. The essence of the human body, blood carries nutrition to the various cells which in turn tune up the organs that keep us alive. In addition, the blood picks up any waste products that need to be eliminated. The Chinese feel that myrrh actually helps the body collect and get rid of the congealed blood of bruises. According to Chinese medicine, the herb's ability to get the blood moving is its main boon to health.

The Chinese go on to say that myrrh soothes pain caused by injury, sores, obstructions, menstruation—essentially any internal pains are made less by its use. The plant product promotes healing, especially in the case of stubborn skin wounds.

Being analytical sorts when it comes to their herbal remedies, the Chinese have investigated myrrh scientifically and found that it lowers serum cholesterol in male rabbits fed high-cholesterol diets. They have also discovered that myrrh stimulates the intestinal tract and has an antifungal action against a number of deadly fungi known to undermine bodily health. Other researchers have proven that myrrh is astringent to the mucous membranes as well as antimicrobial in the test tube. Along these lines, the Indians apply the age-old use of myrrh as a skin healer to the mouth, quite literally. The mouth and throat are, after all, lined with skin, and delicate skin I will add. Ground and applied to the mouth, gums, teeth, and tongue, myrrh is also used in toothpaste, gargles, and sore-throat remedies.

Myrrh can be purchased from most places that deal in herbs, and despite the fact that it is collected by hand in the Middle East, it is reasonably cheap. The gum resin should be a fair yellow color and look almost like lemon drops. The plant has to grow in really dry locations—some of the Southwestern states would be ideal—but getting hold of it is a problem. To my knowledge, the commiphora tree is not sold by any nursery, so we will have to buy this one at the herb seller's.

PLANTAIN

Plantago major

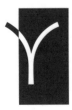ou have seen this one far and wide. Just about everywhere you step, its leathery leaves are not far away. This is the original weed, and I have an admission: until I started rooting around for the 30 top health herbs, I didn't know that plantain was good for anything except the compost heap.

A native of Europe, plantain, like the dandelion, was carried to the four corners in the white man's attempt to own the world. The colonial regimes are gone, but many of the plants they brought with them remain. This common weed, inhabiter of abandoned yards, parking lots, and untended flower gardens, is one of the most widely used medicinal plants. People on every continent collect it and use it to stay well and treat illness. Three generations ago, plantain's use was common knowledge in the United States; today practically no one, and this includes me until very recently, realizes that the plant is anything more than a weed. When folks moved from the countryside to the cities and medically trained doctors replaced family healers, we forgot what we'd known about for years. Until now.

Macer Floridus, which was probably written sometime in the ninth century, gives a good look into early European uses for plantain. In the process of reading through the book, something a sane person who wants to maintain his eyesight would not do, I noticed that the author rarely has much more than a few words to say on each plant. Plantain is a different matter. According to this volume, the plant can be used for: wounds of all sorts including dog bites and scorpion stings, black spots, boils, carbuncles, swellings of the lymph glands, epilepsy, excessive bleeding during menstruation, uterine pains, headaches, coughs, fevers, flu, and sore feet. It is also good for the eyes, gums, and bladder. The list goes on, and on, and on. Who would have thought that such a little weed would actually be so good for so many parts of the body?

Plantago major, or common plantain as we know it, means literally the main solelike plant. The plant's leaves look vaguely like the sole of a shoe, and several names by which it is known in North America, including devil's shoe string, reflect this similarity. In the olden days, when people flocked to the countryside to gather wild herbs for spring tonic, plantain was one of the favorites. A woman from Tennessee declared that the best wild greens were mustard and plantain greens cooked with a ham hock or bacon fat for seasoning. Well, the bacon grease might not be that healthy, but the two other ingredients sure would be.

Have you ever heard the story of the white man's flies? It seems the Indians came to know that the white man was encroaching on their land whenever they saw honey bees, an insect not indigenous to the Americas. The same was true with plantain, which came to be known by the Native Americans as Englishman's foot. It was somewhat of a godsend that the bees and the plantain arrived at the same time, as the leaf of the plantain was used to draw the venom of the bee from its sting. On this the Indian and the white man agreed. The Native Americans grew familiar with the plantain's medicinal properties, and the Delawares used it to treat the summer complaint (that's Victorian for diarrhea).

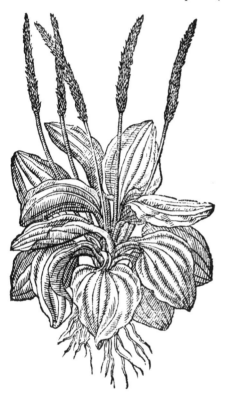

The Pennsylvania Dutch used the juice of the plant to soothe tired and abused feet, treat insect bites, and lessen the pain associated with a bad case of hemorrhoids. The utilitarian people also found that the seeds were effective in getting rid of intestinal worms. In the Louisiana bayou, the fresh leaves were traditionally applied to sores to promote healing, and the dried leaves were put in the linen closet to perfume the contents and keep insects out. An informant in North Carolina said that plantain leaves placed on the wrist of someone with a fever would cure him if the leaves were left on until they were browned by the sick person's heat.

Once again, the Chinese, who are quite familiar with this dooryard weed and use it to treat ailments ranging from rheumatism and infertility to urinary infections and problem deliveries, have scientifically researched some of their claims for it. Like the Delaware Indians, the Chinese say that plantain will take care of a case of the trots. Their studies have proven that plantain does stop diarrhea in children, which can be quite lethal for the little tykes. In addition to tacking down the country notion that plantain relieves the summer complaint, they have backed up the belief that the plant leads to healthier childbirth. The *Materia Medica* mentions a study of women with fetuses in bad positions prior to delivery, in which the use of plantain saw a 90 percent reversal in position— almost all of the women treated had normal presentations at birth.

The plant has received much attention in Burma, where it is used to treat high blood pressure as well as the sores and fevers so common in this steamy part of the world. The Burmese have spent some time looking into plantain's scientific properties, and they have found a number of interesting facts. Plantain in water or alcohol solutions does indeed produce a drop in arterial pressure in dogs. The plant used to treat stomach disorders worldwide has been proven to do just that. The Burmese likewise determined that a substance contained in the plant, plantaglucide, cuts down the ulceration in rats' stomachs by 20 percent. They also found that the substance increases secretion of gastric juices and reduces intestinal contractions, which would indeed alleviate stomach pain.

Time to get personal again, back to the toilet. Plantain contains a lot of mucilage, particularly in its seeds. In the intestinal tract, this substance swells much as gelatin does when you add sugar and water. The effect is that plantain cleans the intestines of toxins and wastes, keeping their function smooth and regular. I keep going back to this because regular elimination is one of the keys to good health.

While we're down there, a delightful home hemorrhoid cream from the gypsies of Eastern Europe includes lard, plantain, and ground ivy. The recipe suggests boiling the ingredients and pressing the resulting mess to get all the plants' power. Once cool, the salve is placed liberally you know where. The Maoris of New Zealand treat the same problem by placing the plant in a steaming pot of water and hanging the afflicted part over the pot: what we like to call a little butt steam. Could be a dangerous proposition, if you ask me. And speaking of parts, Gerard noted that plantain leaves "are singular good to make a water to wash a sore throat or mouth, or the privy parts of a man or woman." Sore privy parts, we all know what that means. Gerard was probably referring to privates plagued with venereal disease. He's not alone in this reference; the plant has long been prized for treating herpes sores (some say it cures them straight away).

PLANTAIN. Here's my favorite way to put plantain's healing power to work in my body. Collect a bag full of fresh plantain, roots and all, take it home, wash it, and trim off the leaves. Heat about three teaspoons of olive oil in a large skillet and add four sliced buds of garlic. When the garlic starts to brown on the edges, toss in the plantain leaves and stir them until they're well wilted. I serve the sauteed leaves with some good whole wheat bread, and believe me, the next day I feel the difference.

As you peruse the world of tonic plants, you will find that there are your middle-of-the-road tonics, and then there are your serious tonics. The serious tonics are the ones, like plantain, which are also listed for treating wasting conditions. This is a good indication of how restorative the plant is. If plantain can reverse the degenerative process for a failing body, imagine what it can do for one in okay condition.

There isn't much sense in growing your own plantain as it's such a readily available weed. Take a walk with a trowel and an old shopping bag, and you will come home with more than you can possibly use. The plant is evergreen, so whenever you decide to make your tonic, plantain will be waiting outside your door, ready to go in your brewing pot.

▼▼▼▼▼▼▼▼▼▼▼▼▼▼▼▼▼▼▼▼

RED CLOVER
Trifolium pratense

n a single conversation I had about clover not so long ago, the people I was chatting with told me that a four-leafed clover is good luck if you place it in your hat or under your pillow and bad luck if you find one and leave it unpicked. I also heard that someone who tries to pick a four-leafed clover in the moonlight will go insane because the good luck of the clover reverses itself.

What is it with the four-leafed clover? Along with losing plant medicine knowledge, we have, for the most part, forgotten plant lore. A couple of hundred years ago, everybody knew the magical powers attributed to plants—what flowers would make your true love love you back, what seed thrown over your shoulder would bring male children or stop the children from coming. Now, when only a few of these folk beliefs remain, it is strange that even the most urbane of us, if asked about four-leafed clover, will quickly affirm that it is good luck.

What's more, this is not a belief held only by North Americans: people everywhere say the same thing. Isn't it peculiar that the odd, four-fingered leaf is considered a wonderful find all over the world? I believe that the litany of magical powers attributed to clovers is due to the undeniable healing powers they exhibit. The conviction that red clover is a tonic to the whole body, strengthening and giving power to the person who drinks it, is almost as universal as the belief in a lucky four-leaf clover.

Whether we admit it or not, the United States is still in many ways a colony of England. We may have severed our political affiliations some time ago, but our cultural affiliations cannot be broken. Clover first came to North America with the English, and their descendants have continued its use. Other British colonies,

Australia, New Zealand, and South Africa included, also received clover and the knowledge surrounding it, and in all those countries today people use clover for healing.

When the English colonists came to North America, they moved from urban settings to a wilderness unlike any they had ever known. It was filled with disease and not a lot of white people. The patches of Englishmen were few and far between, and a settlement with access to a European doctor was a rare phenomenon. People had to take care of themselves.

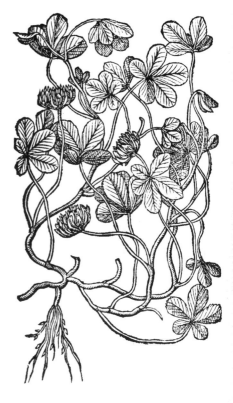

The main "doctor" was usually the mother or the grandmother in the house. It was her responsibility to meet the needs of her sick children or grandchildren, and so mothers made it their business to learn what plants would take a fever away or keep it from coming on in the first place. When a daughter married and went off to an even more remote region where land could be had for the asking, her mother wrote down the remedies that had kept her family alive in a book which the daughter carried with her. In a time when real illness usually meant death, this book was perhaps one of the most sacred items in a woman's possession next to the Bible, for as soon as the babies started coming, their health was dependant on their mother's knowledge of healing plants.

It is during this period in colonial America that we see red clover coming to the fore. Clover, which may be a native of the British Isles, had been known in England as a healing plant and as a blood tonic or purifier since who knows when. Both in the mother country and her colonies, its use went beyond staying well. The notion was that if you were seriously ill, clover could bring you around.

In the absence of modern diagnosis, people looked at disease externally, and they used the term *consumption* to describe what they sometimes saw happening: the body was consumed or eaten away by disease. Sometimes a similar condition was called cancer, and in both cases clover was used to correct the situation.

In some areas, this practice has lingered on into the present. Take a look at this cancer cure from the hills of Tennessee: "Place two to three teaspoons of red clover blossom in one cup of boiling water, steep mixture until a tea is formed. Drink one cup a day." Traditionally, cancer, heart disease, lung disease, and any other serious illnesses were treated with red clover.

Like Englishmen at home, the colonials were tea drinkers. In England, people customarily drank tea in the late afternoon. In the colonies, they were too involved with survival to take a break in the afternoon, so they drank their tea with lunch. Because not everyone could afford the imported beverage, tea substitutes were used, and tea made of dried clover was one of the most popular. Folks also used to make a "spring bracer" or tonic with clover and mint to keep the body in good stead during the all-important planting season. They ate the spring clover greens as salad and pot greens, and made jellies of the red blooms, all to stay healthy.

RED CLOVER. This is the ideal tea-making plant, and what a healing tea it is! Red clover comes into bloom in mid-July, and this is the time to take action. Locate a good clump of blooming clover, cut it to the ground, and carry it home, stems and all. Put a pot of water on the stove, say four cups, and add two cups of clover stems, leaves, and blooms. Once the pot starts to boil, turn off the heat and let the mixture rest for ten minutes or so. Strained and sweetened with honey, this is a tea I would serve to the Garden Club.

Getting back to our goal of making a tonic at home to keep us well, clover was one of the most popular ingredients in tonics in the 1850s. Boiled in water and sweetened with honey, it created the base for many widely sold preparations.

In a book written in 1917, *Health From Field and Forest*, we see clover listed as one of the best blood purifiers, especially in the case of cancer. The volume was essentially a catalogue of items for sale, one of which was that crazy old "Compound No. 7." Though clearly a commercial and not a scholarly undertaking, *Health From Field and Forest* gives you an idea of what people thought about clover at the turn of the century:

Medical scientists have long recognized the value of red clover blossoms as a purifying agent for the blood, particularly in cases of cancerous humors, tumors, carbuncles, and the like, and not only recommend but use them. Knowing this, we have chosen German red-clover, carefully picked and cured in a way to retain its full strength, as a base for our "Red Clover Compound," adding in smaller proportions herbs with qualities like to itself, each serving to bring out and em-

phasize the remedial virtues of the others. Taken freely, as a tea, it purifies the blood and tones up the entire system; and thus by removing the cause, it reaches the very root of the trouble, curing cancers, abscesses, tumors, and other diseases which would never gain a foothold but for an impure condition of the blood. As a remedy for cancer, Compound No. 7 is specific; and as a flesh-producer, if one is for any reason below normal weight, it has no equal. Many use it for this purpose alone. In taking this compound for any of the virulent troubles named one must be persistent and regular. It is not a "cure-while-you-wait" remedy, not a severe purgative which affords seeming relief only to leave the system weakened and debilitated, but a mild, natural tonic, doing its good work steadily and surely without harm or reaction.

It's no wonder that the author specified German red clover. Red clover was, and continues to be, very popular as a healing plant in Germany, and the Mennonites who came to North and South America to escape religious persecution in that country brought this information with them. To this day in the American communities, they use red clover, known as *rhoda glae blumma*, to treat whooping cough, croup, and cancer of the stomach, and its roots to treat diphtheria.

Half a world away, the Chinese likewise revere clover, *hsun tsao*, as a tonic, and they draw the sap to treat colds and influenza. At one time in Chinese history, the dried plant was burned at altars as an incense. If you wanted to have a chat with the gods, the way to invite them down was to light a little clover. It was also worn in the girdle to expel any bad vibes that might be hanging around. Contemporary Chinese researchers don't have much to say about bad vibes, but they have proven that red clover kills certain viral and fungal infections, has estrogenlike functions, and is an antispasmodic and expectorant.

Red clover is another one of our tonic ingredients that needn't be bought or raised. Take a car trip out to the countryside in July and collect the red blossoms with wild abandon—any country road will provide you with more than you could ever need. One cautionary note: insects that sting, otherwise known as bees, are fond of clover, and are apt to be near. Give each clover plant a good shake before you start collecting, or you are likely to get a sharp surprise on one of your fingers which could conclude your venture prematurely. When you get your cache home, spread the blossoms out over a large table to dry. This should take place within a week. Once they are crisply dried, put them in sealed jars, and store the jars in a dark location until you are ready to make your tonic.

▼▼▼▼▼▼▼▼▼▼▼▼▼▼▼▼▼▼▼▼▼▼▼▼

SAINT-JOHN'S-WORT
Hypericum perforatum

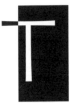he many folk names for Saint-John's-wort—balm of warrior's wounds, the devil's scourge, touch and heal, and witches' herb, to mention a few—give a healthy hint as to what the country people felt about this plant. I think my favorite name is the Lord God's wonder plant. Can you imagine having to spit out that name every time you wanted someone to hand you some Saint-John's-wort? All my research indicates, however, that doing so would be worth the trouble.

Saint-John's-wort has enjoyed a reputation as a wound herb since the fifth century, B.C. Dioscorides, Paul of Aegina, Pliny, and Galen all referred to the plant, which is said to relieve excessive pain, remove the effects of shock, and have a tonic effect on the mind and body. As such, it is an especially valuable treatment for the pain which follows an operation.

From ancient times, Saint-John's-wort was known as a miracle healer, and, like many health-giving plants, it earned a reputation for magical properties as well. As one of its folk names suggests, "witches' herb" was popular with practitioners of witchcraft, perhaps because when its flowers are pressed with cooking oil, they produce a blood-red substance. And I mean to say blood red. The leaves are marked with spots the color of dried blood. The red juice of the crushed flowers was believed to be the blood of Saint John the Baptist, and the flowers were traditionally gathered on the Eve of Saint John's Day, June 24. The so-called "witches' blood" obtained from the plant was an important ingredient in love potions and conjuring spells from the days of the early Greeks onward.

There is not one Saint-John's-wort, but several, and almost every continent has been blessed with its own variety. Used to maintain health since antiquity, the plants are now finding a place in the modern medicinal arena. Contemporary herbalists are using the plant in treating AIDS and other immunity-suppressed conditions, so there's a good chance that we will be hearing more about Saint-John's-wort in the coming years.

Earlier herbalists and healers have had a lot to say on the subject. In 1597, our friend Gerard noted:

Saint John's wort with his flowers and seed boiled and drunken, provoketh urine, and is right good against the stone in the bladder, and stoppeth the laske. The leaves stamped are good to be laid upon burnings, scaldings, and all wounds; and also for rotten and filthy ulcers.

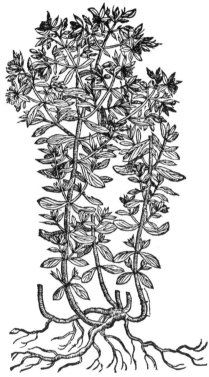

The *Lewis Materia Medica*, compiled in 1799, adds that the plant was useful for "maniacal disorders." In fact, "it has been reckoned of such efficacy in the later as to have thence received the name fuga daemonum [go away, demons]. It has also been recommended internally for wounds, bruises, ulcers, spitting blood, bloody urine, agues, and worms." As I certainly have my share of unwanted demons, it's nice to know that the plant will take care of them while it is making my body strong.

A North American observer named Rafinesque remarked in 1830 that the leaves could be used to relieve diseases of the breast and that a syrup of sage and Saint-John's-wort was useful in cases of croup, colic, and vomiting. By 1868, the plant had a listing in the Canadian Pharmacopeia.

In 1892, a scientist wrote of Saint-John's-wort:

The great use of hypericum in wounds where the nerves are involved to any extent is the rightful discovery of the true science of medicine, many cases of injury to the cranium and spinal column are reported benefitted by its use, and every homeopathic physician of at least three months practice can attest to its merits.

In 1992, the plant is still considered supreme among homeopaths, but nobody else in the United States seems to use it for squat. Most of us can't recognize it if it's under our noses, let alone know how to use it. Cattle and sheep ranchers in the West are familiar with it because Saint-John's-wort causes sensitivity to light, and the animals that eat a lot of it get killer sunburns. (Once again, this is an herb where a little goes a long way; it can make people as well as livestock more sensitive to the sun.) As a result of this characteristic, both the ranchers and the government are trying to eradicate the "useless" weed.

Okay, it's time to re-remember the plant all witches love. To do so, let's go overseas where folks still recognize it.

SAINT-JOHN'S-WORT. This makes a sensational healing ointment. Take four cups of fresh or dried Saint-John's-wort and four cups of olive oil, and grind them in the food processor. Let the mixture sit for a week in a covered glass container in a sunny window. Then pour the liquid through a spaghetti strainer and into mason jars. Once called dragon's blood, the preparation actually does take on a bright red color, a tiny bit of which is transferred to the skin. Being a gardener, I am forever scratching myself and irritating my skin. When this happens, on goes the dragon's blood.

In Ukrainian folk medicine, Saint-John's-wort is a leading home remedy, especially for kidney problems and ailments of the digestive tract ranging from stomachaches to stomach cancer, and oddly enough including both constipation and diarrhea. It is also used for respiratory, metabolic, and gynecological diseases, as well as infectious ones. The Ukrainians wash both their hair and their wounds with various parts of the plant; it's even recommended for the treatment of cattle that have been bitten by mad dogs.

The villagers also use Saint-John's-wort as a tonic to ensure good strength for the long days of labor at harvest time. The feeling is that the plant makes you strong and more able to handle your work. Does this sound like something you might want to have, strength to do the things you need to do?

In Ireland, Saint-John's-wort is associated with the Blessed Virgin and Saint Columcille as well as Saint John. The plant was recommended by the chief herbalist in County Waterford as an excellent remedy for an airy fit. In case you're not up on Irish terminology, an airy fit is a little spell of lunacy, something which tends to happen from time to time to most of us living in the modern world.

In China, *Hypericum chinense*, or *ssu tsao* as it is called, is both an ornamental and a medicinal plant. Unlike other members of the species which lack in this department, the flowers of the Chinese variety are said to be lovely. The plant is used as an astringent and is also prescribed for diseases resulting from fouled water sources and snake bites. If you are sick, *si zao* is thought to alter that state

Thirty Plants That Can Save Your Life!

even though the preferred way of taking the plant is with a sip of wine and a touch of powdered centipede. Yuck.

Leave it to the Chinese to check things out scientifically, and here is what they learned about one of their local Saint-John's-worts: Japanese Saint-John's-wort, along with several other hypericum species, has been shown to have anti-tumor activity in animals. At least 17 species of hypericum demonstrate in vitro antibacterial properties. Other hypericum species display in vitro antifungal activity, and seven species are reported to elicit antiviral effects in vitro. In addition, extracts of *Hypericum perforatum* have produced antidiarrheal, sedative, antitumor, and diuretic results.

So there you have it. Saint-John's-wort is a serious ingredient in our tonic mixture. In getting hold of your raw material, you have a couple of options: you can buy it, you can collect it, or you can grow it. It is readily available at natural food stores, or you can go out and collect it. The plant is best collected when it's in bloom, and you'll want to keep the stems, leaves, and flowers attached. They can be dried in a shady location for later use or tossed into the witches' pot fresh.

If you decide you would like to grow some of your own, this is a smart thing to do as no garden plant could be easier to deal with. Get a start from the garden center or from a friend and haul it in. Saint-John's-wort likes both full sun and total shade. It will be more than happy to take over whatever space you have for it and grow like bananas, so to speak. The plant makes a pretty intense ground cover once it gets started, but because you will be picking so much of it, you don't need to worry about losing garden control.

▼▼▼▼▼▼▼▼▼▼▼▼▼▼▼▼▼▼▼▼▼▼▼▼

SARSAPARILLA
Smilax ornata

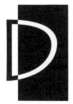
id you ever wonder why old-fashioned drugstores had soda counters and fountains? Many years ago, in the days when everybody took tonics, the tonics were often made by druggists. They would collect tonic plants and brew them into a syrup which was then sweetened with honey or sugar. Formerly, people bought tonic syrups from the druggist and mixed their tonic syrup with water at home. At the turn of the

century, carbonated water came into vogue, and the druggists began offering their brand tonics mixed with soda water right at the drugstore. One of the most popular tonics of the day was root beer. The base of root beer was made of ginger root, sassafras root, and sarsaparilla, and to this pharmacists added their own favorite herbs. But that was then—today's root beer is usually artificially flavored.

Sarsaparilla is furnished by the root of a climbing plant of the genus Smilax, 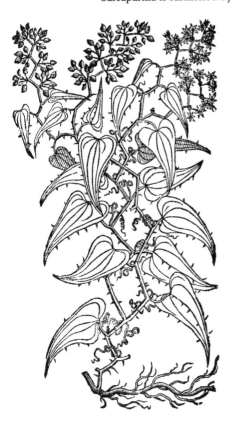 which prevails over the northern part of South America, the whole of Central America, the west coast of Mexico, and up and down the East Coast of the United States. While there are a number of different sarsaparillas used in medicine, all reputedly have about the same health-giving properties. The plant was said to have been introduced to Seville about 1536 from "New Spain" and Honduras. Pedro de Cieze de Leon's *Chronicle of Peru*, written in 1553, mentions sarsaparilla as growing in South America, where the Spaniard had observed it as early as 1533. He found it to be one of the most excellent New World remedies he had encountered and considered it particularly good at treating syphilis and acute debility. The Spanish called it *zarza parilla*, which was altered to create the English word *sarsaparilla*.

Writing in 1559, Girolamo Cardano of Milan deemed it the supreme blood purifier and body enhancer. When the British arrived on American shores, they too ran into sarsaparilla and valued it as highly as the Spanish had.

Because the plant is indigenous to the Americas, most early mentions of it come from contacts colonials made with the Native Americans. In 1624, Sagard reported its use among the Huron tribe for healing sores, ulcers, and wounds. In 1708, Sarrazin-Vaillant wrote of the northern sarsaparilla, "The plant passed here for sarsaparilla because its root is something like it and has the same virtues almost as powerfully. I treated a patron who two years ago was cured of dropsy by using a drink of the root of this plant." Carver had even more to say about sarsaparilla in 1778:

The root of this plant, which is the most estimable part of it, is about the size of a goose quill, and runs in different directions, twined and crooked, to a great length in the ground, and from the principal stele of it springs many smaller fibers, all of which are tough and flexible, the bark of the root, which alone should be used in medicine, is of a bitterish flavor, but aromatic, it is deservedly esteemed for its medicinal virtues, being a gentle sudorifin and very powerful in attenuating the blood when impeded by gross humors.

The Native Americans felt pretty strongly about sarsaparilla, believing it to be the supreme spring and blood tonic. The Chippewa, Meskwaki, Ojibwa, Potawatomi, and the Tete de Boule tribes all reported to the colonials that when an illness threatened to turn into consumption, sarsaparilla should be taken immediately. The belief was that any weakness could be turned into strength with the addition of some sarsaparilla. By the mid-1800s, its use had caught on among white physicians who, according to Gunn, prescribed it as a treatment "in constitutional diseases, such as scrofula, syphilis, skin diseases, and where an alterative and purifying medicine is needed." By the year 1868, the plant was esteemed highly enough that it was included in an official list of Canadian medicinal plants.

The root beer served at so many drugstores was first called New Orleans Mead, presumably due to its popularity among Louisiana's Cajuns and Creoles. In case you are interested in making a little for yourself, here is a recipe from the 1876 *Canadian Pharmacy*:

SARSAPARILLA. Homemade root-beer syrup takes gourmet into a new dimension: guests get a kick out of the flavor option for their drinks, and nothing could be easier for the host. Take one cup of grated ginger root, two cups of sassafras root, two cups of sarsaparilla root, and one teaspoon of ginseng root, and place them in a big pot with one gallon of water. Let the mixture boil for a half hour, or until the water has reduced down by half. Pour the remaining liquid through a spaghetti strainer into big pot number two. Depending on how healthy you feel, add either five cups of sugar or five cups of honey. Bring the liquid back to a high boil and pour it into jars. I serve two tablespoons in each tumbler of club soda, but the exact amount is a matter of personal preference.

8 ounces of sarsaparilla, licorice, cassia, and ginger. 2 ounces of cloves, 3 ounces of coriander seed, boil for fifteen minutes in eight gallons of water, let it stand until cold. Then strain through flannel and add to it in the soda fountain, syrup

12 pints, honey 4 pints, tincture of ginger 4 ounces, and solution of citric acid 4 ounces.

The main ingredient, as you can see, was sarsaparilla. For all we know, it may still be an important component of commercial root beers, but there's no way to tell because contemporary soda manufacturers refuse to reveal their recipes. Luckily, the Choctaw Indians were more forthcoming. They considered sarsaparilla the best available general tonic, and they told the Creole country doctors about it. According to Zora Neale Hurston's *Mules and Men*, root doctors in the bayou also used it in prescriptions for those who suffered from venereal diseases and "lost minds." And to this day, country folk will tell you that the root is number one for blood cleansing and strengthening.

Though root beer may have started in Louisiana, it caught on quickly throughout the United States, and a number of similar products were offered up for sale. The Shakers advertised their "Compound Concentrated Syrup of Sarsaparilla" in 1837 with an assertion that:

This medicine, taken in doses of an once, 4 or 5 times a day will fulfill every indication that the boasted panaceas and catholicons can perform; is free from the mercurial poisons such nostrums contain; and is much more safe and efficient as a medicine for cleansing and purifying the blood.

Like the Native Americans, the Shakers believed that when an alterative was needed, this was the plant. Whatever ailed you would be taken away with the use of sarsaparilla, or the syrup thereof. For years pharmacists from coast to coast agreed, and used it in their pet formulas for tonics. We will too.

You can buy sarsaparilla root from your local herb seller, who gets it from the Caribbean Islands, Mexico, or South America, or you can gather it yourself. The North American wild stock has been pretty hard hit in the past century, but it still can be found in patches up and down the East Coast and working towards the West. I have never heard of sarsaparilla's being planted in the garden, but that's not to say that it couldn't be done.

▼▼▼▼▼▼▼▼▼▼▼▼▼▼▼▼▼▼▼▼▼▼

SAW PALMETTO

Sarenoa serrulata

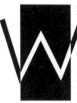hen I set out to compile the list of the most widely used tonic plants, there were very few surprises as I already had at least a passing acquaintance with most of the plants. This was not the case with saw palmetto. Frankly, I had never even heard of it before its name started popping up in the volumes I read. Though its story is not as international as some of the other plants, I think it deserves the place it has won in this book.

I'm often asked how on earth people learned what plants were good for what condition. It's a good question, and saw palmetto provides a perfect example of how the process works. It can be summed up in one word: observation.

Saw palmetto grows along the southeastern coast of the United States where it forms a palmetto scrub for hundreds of miles along the coastline from Georgia to Florida. Rarely more than a few feet high, the plants rarely amount to much in size, but their fan-shaped, glaucous leaves are so dense that a stand of these palms is virtually impossible for human beings to pass through and certainly less than pleasant to clear. To the region's early settlers, they were a pain in the butt.

As the settlers cut down parts of the scrub for pastureland, they noticed an interesting thing: their animals would lean over the fences to get at the berries of this palm. What's more, the animals that ate the black fruit were healthier than those that did not. Before you know it, the settlers were purposefully feeding their animals palmetto berries to improve their health, and in time, they decided that saw palmetto might do the same for themselves. And it did.

In 1877, a Dr. Reed took the process one step further when he researched the settlers' practice and published an article describing his findings in the *Medical Brief* of St. Louis. Entitled "A New Remedy," Reed's article was reprinted in July 1879 in a publication called *New Preparations*. The volume also included a piece from the *Medical Brief* written by Dr. I. J. M. Goss, then of Marietta, Georgia, who had drawn similar conclusions about the plant. From this point, the tonic makers got wind of saw palmetto and began including it in lots of recipes for staying well.

The doctors of the day found the fruit to be a nutritive tonic, an effective diuretic, and a mild sedative. It was recommended for all wasting diseases, and was said to have a marked effect on the glandular systems. Most notably, it had an ability to increase flesh rapidly.

Although saw palmetto's health-building powers came as news to the settlers, the natives of the region knew all about them. The Seminole Indians apparently ground the berries into a nutritious flour. They are also said to have used an

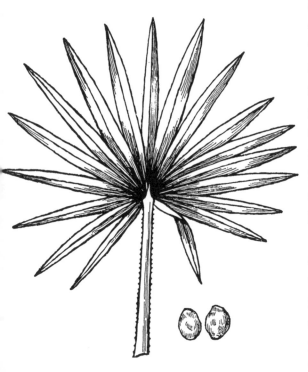

infusion for stomachache and dysentery. The inner bark of the trunk was used as a pack for snake bites, bug bites, and skin ulcers. Dried fruits were believed useful for indigestion, respiratory infections, and catarrhal irritation. One of the more noteworthy claims that comes to us from the Native Americans concerns the plant's ability to enlarge breasts and sexual desire.

The root doctors of the Louisiana bayou also were well acquainted with the palmetto. Descending from French, Indian, and African stock, these inheritors of the local plant wisdom used palmetto berries to treat syphilis and other infectious diseases. One recipe calls for red oak bark, palmetto root, fig root, two pinches of alum, nine drops of turpentine, and two quarts of water, with all ingredients boiled down to one quart to be taken one half a cup at a time. While the plant's ability to bolster the body would make it helpful in the case of many infectious diseases, curing syphilis is a tall order.

Still the local doctors were so impressed with the changes that occurred when they administered saw palmetto berries to ailing patients that they called for further research on the secret substance contained therein. Sadly, this research has yet to be done.

Despite being overlooked by the scientific community, the plant continues to be used by the natural healing community. There the berries remain a hot commodity, collected in the southern states and sold to natural food stores and to people practicing old-time healing techniques.

Many of the berries find their way into modern tonics offered for sale at health food stores. Pick up a bottle of any "vitality formula," and there you will see the berry in question, listed as plain as day. I was at the gym the other day, chatting with the guy next to me in the locker room. He had muscles that don't even exist on my body, and he was chirping away happily about the natural tea that made all those ripples possible. A quick read of the ingredient panel disclosed none other than saw palmetto berries. It seems that body builders world 'round are now discovering what the palmetto pioneers found out so many years back.

SAW PALMETTO. *Saw palmetto is definitely a tonic plant (this is my way of preparing the adventurer for a less-than-satisfying tongue experience). I'm not crazy about the taste, but saw palmetto is considered the health food of the prostrate, and that's something most of us boys want to keep fit as a fiddle. To make a healthful decoction, take one half cup of saw palmetto berries and four cups of water and bring the combination to a high boil. Let the mixture rest for a half an hour, add one tablespoon of it (discarding the pulp) to two cups of boiling water, and drink away.*

Unlike the chemical steroids previously and currently used by narcissists in search of the perfect build, saw palmetto berries do not damage sexual function. To the contrary, the saw palmetto is an aphrodisiac of some note, held to improve prostrate function, which in turn improves male sexual performance. And, of course, the Native American women used them to increase their bust size. So what's sauce for the goose is also sauce for the gander.

Modern herbalists have learned that these same berries work on head colds and all their accompanying symptoms. It appears that a tea made of the berries somehow kicks the air passages back into shape and tones the lungs while it's at it. In addition, saw palmetto is used as both a sedative and a stimulant.

From the moment that first Carolina planter noticed how big his pigs got on a diet of saw palmetto berries, people have used them to treat wasting conditions, to rejuvenate an old or ill body, and to beef up a healthy one. The underlying theme is that saw palmetto strengthens. Of course, the downside is that you might accidentally become incredibly muscle-bound. But for most of us, that's a risk worth taking.

SCHIZANDRA

Schisandra chinensis

Our next ingredient, schizandra, has been a well-kept Asian secret, but not for much longer. I have a feeling that once people start discovering its virtues, the imports from China will go straight through the ceiling. I don't have much cocktail party trivia to amuse you with about this one. However, it is such a great plant that I had to include it in our tonic. Take a look at some schizandra facts.

The fruit of the schizandra has been proven to stimulate the spinal cord and brain and to strengthen and quicken the reflexes; when people were fed it, they 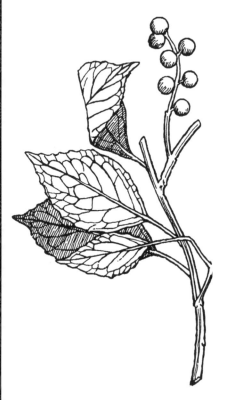 worked better and more efficiently. Though stimulating, it does not have the twitchy side effects of caffeine. It wouldn't surprise me if major corporations started dropping the berries in their water coolers.

It has also been shown to stimulate breathing by affecting the central nervous system. The exact process is not yet understood, but it works so powerfully that the plant is used in morphine overdoses to counteract the respiratory paralysis that often leads to death in such cases. With a 76 percent success rate in treating certain types of hepatitis, schizandra has likewise proven an effective cure for chronic liver diseases.

When taken intravenously, it decreases blood pressure, and in alcoholic solutions, it acts as a vasodilator. It has been shown to stimulate rabbits' uteruses before, during, and after pregnancy. Specifically, it strengthens rhythmic contractions, and as such, it is used in promoting and procuring healthy labors.

What's more, schizandra aids in the digestion and absorption of nutrients into the body. It increases visual acuity and the field of vision as well as the ability to discern different sorts of touches. In short, it improves the sensory perceptions. It also increases people's ability to deal effectively with stress and improves their endurance. Once again, this was proven with mice in a lap pool. Taking the plant makes animals and people alike better able to deal with their environment.

There are two kinds of schizandra plants, one producing red berries and the other black. The red berries are the fruits you see at the Chinese herbalist's shop; the black ones rarely make it out of Asia.

The fruits are said to have five distinct flavors: sweet, sour, pungent, bitter, and salty. This feature of the plant gave rise to its name in Chinese, *wu wei tsu*, the five-flavored plant. Now, back to my theory that all tonic plants show off their specialness in some special way. Lemons are sour, dates are sweet, and any fruit with five flavors is mighty odd in my book. This fact alone would have hinted to early observers that something was up with schizandra.

As schizandra is a Chinese plant, to understand its medicinal use we must first learn through which channel the plant enters the body. If you guessed the lung and kidney channels, you were correct. Schizandra first appeared in the *Divine Husbandman's Classic of the Materia Medica*, which is to say that it has been around for thousands of years. The plant is used to treat a lot of different things, including coughs, premature ejaculation, chronic dysentery, and insomnia.

SCHIZANDRA. I'm not sure that the Chinese masters would appreciate my use of schizandra, but they don't have to—I am the one who has to eat it. I make what I like to call schizandra marmalade. Take four cups of schizandra berries and four cups of honey and cook the mixture over low heat until the berries fall apart. Because the combination is highly sugared, stir constantly so that it doesn't burn. Once the berries have softened to a mush, take the marmalade off the heat, put it in jars, and keep it in the refrigerator for smearing on toast.

The thing I want to zero in on about schizandra is its role as what the Chinese call an adaptogen. This is the concept in Chinese medicine that Westerners have the hardest time grasping because the adaptogen is an herb category we don't even have. Adaptogens are plants that help you adapt to your environment. Let's take another adaptogen, garlic, as an example. People eat garlic in hot countries so that the heat doesn't make them sick; in high altitudes, it's consumed to make breathing easier. It is also used to kill the unfamiliar bacteria folks encounter on trips. Garlic helps you adjust to any environment you happen to be in, and schizandra does the same thing. In essence, all of our tonic plants are adaptogens. That's what preventative medicine is all about, helping the body to cope so that it never gets ill.

SELF-HEAL PRUNELLA

Prunella vulgaris

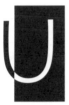

Unlike our last tonic plant, self-heal is no secret—it's used on every continent human beings call home. The fact that this plant is also known as heal-all and cure-all should give you some insight into what people have found to be true of it. They don't call it sometimes-heal, or might-heal, or every-once-in-a-while-heal, they call it heal-all.

Self-heal is a mint relation, and as with all the other mints, if you plant it once, you never have to plant it again. Incredibly vigorous, the plant spreads by underground stems that shoot out in every direction once the first root is stuck in the ground. If there is anything to the doctrine of signatures, prunella should make anyone who takes it into his or her body stronger than an ox.

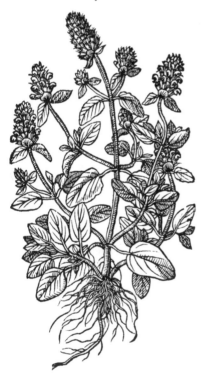

In the southern United States, ground-hog plantain, or square weed as it is called, is collected in the spring as a tonic plant. It is also eaten as a spinach substitute, prepared in a big pot with a piece of hog meat by cooks who follow the traditional southern style or with a little vegetable oil by more modern cooks concerned with the bad publicity animal fats have received in recent years.

In China, where, as it does worldwide, the plant grows great guns, it is called *hsia-ku-tsao* and is widely used as a tonic. The Chinese, who collect the plant as it spikes into bloom, take the lower leaves and flower heads from it to treat fevers and rheumatism. They also use the leaves and flower heads as an alterative, a substance which helps the body change from a state of sickness to one of health. When self-heal is taken in tea, the Chinese feel that the plant can keep the entire body well. It is said to assist liver function, resulting in bright, clear eyes. As such, self-heal is used to treat patients suffering from eye or liver trouble. It is also used to treat lumps in the neck and swollen glands. This ties in with its use as an immunity booster: when your body gets run down, those lymph glands swell right up.

Knowing the Chinese use self-heal as an alterative, we should not be surprised to learn that the plant has an antibiotic effect. Experiments indicate that self-heal has broad antimicrobial powers and also kills many pathogenic fungi, the kind that attack the body and do you no good.

Self-heal is well known in Europe, and our friend Gerard had additional uses to list, noting that "the decoction of Prunell made with wine or water, doth joine together and make whole and sound all wounds, both inward and outward, even as Bugle doth." His reference to the plant's ability to make things whole after the body has suffered both external and internal injuries is consistent with other European sources: as the name says, the plant helps healing. Gerard also wrote of prunella's potency as a headache treatment when "bruised with oil of roses and vinegar, and laid to the forepart of the head," and he recommended the plant "against the infirmities of the mouth, and especially the ruggedness, blackness, and dryness of the tongue, with a kind of swelling in the same. It is an infirmitie amongst soldiers that lie in campe."

SELF-HEAL PRUNELLA. My favorite way to use this pleasant-tasting plant is whole, in a fresh or wilted salad. I grow self-heal prunella in my garden for a constant source, so I toss a few leaves in the salad bowl whenever I like. Self-heal is especially good with watercress, pears, and raisins. For a delicious wilted salad, saute six sliced garlic cloves in olive oil until they are brown around the edges. Then add eight cups of self-heal leaves, stir rapidly until the leaves are wilted, remove the salad from the heat, and serve.

I'll tell you one thing: if I ever woke up and found I had a black tongue, I would get real nervous real fast. Having your tongue turn black is Mother Nature's way of saying that you need to work on your health regime. Gerard's reference to soldiers "that lie in campe" is significant. Soldiers live in close quarters, and when a sickness hits the barracks, it spreads like wildfire, kind of like a cold running through the office. Self-heal has a widespread reputation for keeping people well during an outbreak of infectious disease. This, of course, makes it perfect for life in the modern world.

In colonial America, self-heal should have been called heal- anything-you've-got, as its uses were incredibly diverse. It was used to treat sore throats, stomach cramps, and urinary and liver problems. It was also prescribed to kill worms and to help folks who suffered from fits. It's main use though was as a tonic.

The Shakers sold lots of self-heal to treat internal bleeding, sore throats, and cankers in the mouth. Also in agreement with Gerard, they believed that self-heal was good for black tongues and cold sores. The gypsies of Eastern Europe, who gave a double ditto on self-heal's ability to cure sore throats, used it as an ingredient in their medicine show tonics for that problem.

In New Zealand the plant gets wide use as a first aid ointment—the ground plant is applied to cuts, wounds, bruises, and sores that won't heal. The Kiwis are not alone in the thought that whatever the plant touches heals a lot faster than it otherwise would. Like Gerard, they say that putting the juice of its leaves and flowers on the temples will take care of a headache in short order.

Most would agree that the heart is an organ we would like to keep pumping away, trouble-free. Self-heal is featured in an Irish heart-disease treatment called Cailleach's Tea. Chinese researchers have found the plant to be an effective remedy for hypertension, a fact which would indeed make Cailleach's Tea useful for someone whose heart troubles stem from high blood pressure.

"Heal-all" is a steep claim, but even if it's only partially true, we would all be better off with self-heal prunella in our tonic pot. As I've already mentioned, growing it, or more accurately letting it grow itself, is no problem. Stick some in the ground and stand back. When you are harvesting self-heal for the tonic pot, cut the plant as it breaks into bloom, trimming it off one inch above the roots. The plant won't mind—as a matter of fact, this gives it an incentive to grow more.

▼▼▼▼▼▼▼▼▼▼▼▼▼▼▼▼▼▼▼▼

YELLOW DOCK

Rumex crispus

Dock plant is a common weed. You can find it growing all over the place, most often, as the name indicates, beside a dock. To positively identify yellow dock, turn to the back of a commercial herbicide package—this dear plant is usually pictured among the intended victims. Most modern gardeners think of yellow dock the same way they do dandelion and burdock, as a useless weed. They're wrong. The plant is anything but useless and deserves a more respectful title than "weed."

It is fair to say that yellow dock is far from decorative. It has evergreen leaves and a flower that looks like anything but. The seed mass is a rust color, reminiscent of a huge wad of tobacco. So, not everyone can be pretty. But as I like to say, don't judge a plant by its listing on the back of a can of weed killer!

Like dandelion and burdock, yellow dock was once a very popular spring tonic plant. In many parts of the world, people will tell you that meat prepared with dock cooks much faster than normal. I would say this is some special feature. All you folks on the run might want to let this plant stay on in your backyards for those occasions when you have to snap together a quick dinner.

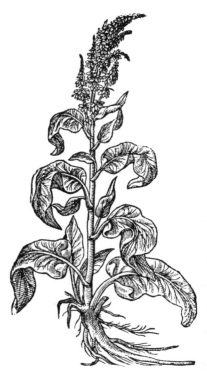

During North America's colonial days, one plant that came as a real surprise to the Europeans, and an unpleasant surprise at that, was poison ivy. The old-time treatment for a bad case of poison ivy (and as these were people who went to the bathroom in the woods, they got some really serious cases) was yellow dock boiled with vinegar and applied to the sores.

Dock leaves were likewise used to treat scrofulous sores, sore eyes, and glandular swellings. To cure itchy skin, they were bruised, mixed with butter, lard, or cream, and placed on the problem area. The colonials also used the plant as a treatment for the runs, which was a common problem in the New World. They believed that if the plant was eaten on a regular basis, it would improve the eyesight as well.

The Mennonites were quite familiar with this weed. They called it *halwer gaul* and considered it the best blood purifier on the planet. Accordingly, they used it to treat liver problems of all kinds along with the skin problems resulting from poor liver function, and still do to this day. It's interesting to note that Arab physicians recommend the same plant for hepatitis and poor digestion, and they are a long, long way from the Pennsylvania Dutch Country.

Not surprisingly for a plant with such widely recognized powers in aiding the liver, dock leaves were mixed with elderberry leaves to draw the poison out of rattlesnake or copperhead bites. Like echinacea, dock was a traditional snake plant, thought to help the body rid itself of venom.

In 1898, a homeopathic doctor had a few choice words to toss in on this topic: "There are three localities in which this remedy acts very markedly, respiratory organs, bowels, and skin....There is perhaps no remedy under which the sensibility of the mucous membrane of the larynx and trachea become more exalted than this one."

So up to this point, yellow dock is good for the blood, liver, stomach, skin, and the respiratory tract. Could there be more? You know that the answer is yes.

Good old Gerard recommended yellow dock as a key ingredient in a tonic which he claimed "cureth the dropsie, the yellow jaunders, all manner of itch, scabes, breaking out, and manginesse of the whole body... purifieth the blood from all corruption; prevaileth against the green sickness very greatly, and...maketh young wenches to look faire and cherrie like." I think my favorite line from that passage is "maketh young wenches to look faire and cherrie like." I wonder if Gerard called all women wenches. I think not. But if you want your wench to look fine, or if you are a wench yourself and would like to look the same, this is the plant for you.

YELLOW DOCK. This is another plant with a squarely tonic flavor, which I take for tonic purposes whenever I feel run down. Boil one teaspoon of yellow dock root in one cup of water for one minute, let the tea rest for five, and then down it goes. Some people eat the leaves in salads, but the times I have done this, I have always come to the same conclusion: there's a reason yellow dock is not sold in frozen packages next to the broccoli and spinach. I much prefer a cup of dock tea to a bowlful of the nasty-tasting greens.

Various cultures around the world have used yellow dock for ailments ranging from cancer and tuberculosis to syphilis and leprosy to ringworm and hemorrhoids. In India, they even use the root juice for toothaches and the powdered roots for gingivitis and as a dentifrice. In what is perhaps a two-for-one deal, the Maoris of New Zealand chew the leaf first and then apply it to wounds, which they claim then heal without visible scars. The overall universal conclusion is that this plant is one of the best.

On a scientific level, researchers feel that herbal extracts may inhibit escherichia, salmonella, and staphylococcus. In other words, yellow dock contains several antimicrobial agents capable of killing off nasty little bacteria.

Now this is a plant you can buy, collect, or let grow in your garden whenever it shows up, which it certainly will. The evergreen leaves and the root are the parts to use in your tonic, so gather them when you want. Remember, as with all our tonic ingredients, the rule is: the fresher, the better.

Thirty Plants That Can Save Your Life!

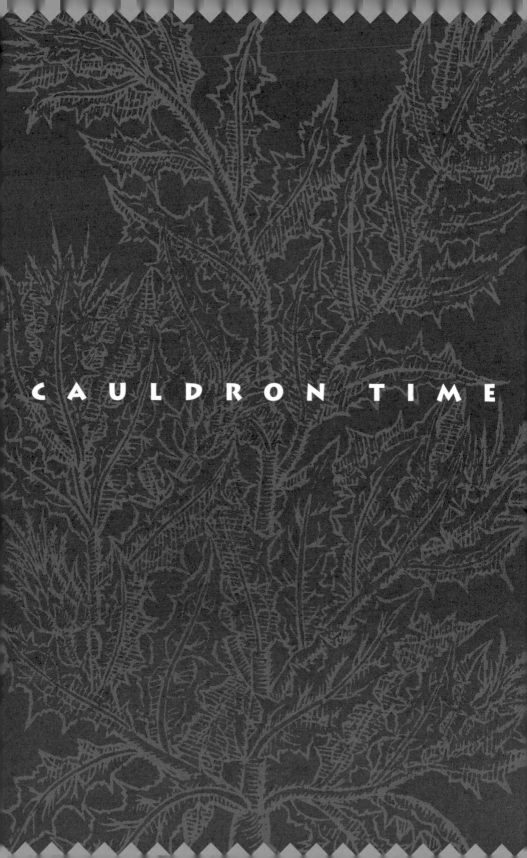

CAULDRON TIME

ow you have the list of ingredients we will use to make our tonic: 30 plants that could clearly save your life. It's a pretty impressive group, if you ask me, but what you've read about them is the tip of the iceberg. If you are interested in learning more, there is no shortage of information on these and other special plants. For a great general introduction to the subject, go to the library and find *A Modern Herbal* by Maud Grieve (Dover, 1971). It's a two-volume reference book no home should be without.

Our next step is to mix the plants up and make a product that we can use on a daily basis to stay well. To do so, we will have to obtain all 30. If you are buying them, buy them. If you are growing them, go out and cut them, and if you are collecting them, get your boots on and gather them. The recipe for what I like to call "Turbo Tonic" looks like this:

2 tablespoons of each and every herb (except barberry, juniper, honey, dates, and figs)

½ teaspoon barberry

½ teaspoon juniper

4 cups honey

4 cups dates

4 cups figs

3 gallons mineral or bottled water

In the way of supplies, you will need a big pot (something large enough to hold four gallons) and one box of quart-sized mason jars.

With all the ingredients and supplies at hand, it's time to move on to the next step. Put ¼ cup of each herb, excluding the honey, dates, and figs, into your pot. Then add the mineral water and place the pot on the stove top on high. Stirring from time to time and mashing the herbs as much as possible, let the mixture boil until about one third of the water has boiled off.

Turn off the heat. When the mixture is cool enough to work with, pour it through a sieve, keeping the liquid and discarding the herbs. Their magic is now contained in the water, and this is what we want to use. Put the herbed water back into the pot.

Now chop the figs and dates to a pulp. It's easiest to use a food processor, but you can also do it by hand with a knife. When the healing fruits have been worked to a mushlike consistency, add them to the pot. Bring the mixture to a second boil until all the fruit has dissolved. Remove it from the heat, and when it is cool, add the honey. Again, allow the mixture to boil for 30 minutes, stirring all the while. With the addition of the sugary fruits and honey, the tonic is likely to burn if not constantly attended. The message is: the last half hour is critical, and you have to keep an eye on the stove top at all times.

Once the cooking is complete, pour the mixture in the mason jars, twist the seals, and stand back. Once cool, it is ready for use.

On my last trip to Spain, as I interviewed men and women in their 80s who were still working the fields, I discovered one thing: these people take their tonics every day for a lifetime. They don't take them for a few weeks and give up; they take them over a long period of time. So plan to continue making and using your tonic. Most of the tonics from days gone by were taken one tablespoon every morning with breakfast, and this is probably the best course of action.

I'm telling you right now that the "Turbo Tonic" won't win any prizes in the taste department, and that no tonic works overnight. They work gradually, slowly, so if you don't notice a difference immediately, don't give up. If this slow approach doesn't appeal to you, understand that you are your own worst enemy. There is no quick fix, no instant cure. Centuries of experience tell us that the patient and continued use of these plants will lead to a long and healthy life.

Being a realist, I recognize that getting all 30 plants in the same room at the same time may represent too formidable a task for those of you who are short on time, so I have put together some quicker tonic recipes for your convenience. The "Turbo Tonic" is a great all-purpose tonic; these others are a little more specific. Read the descriptions and see if any of them strike a cord with you and your health record.

FOR THE BOYS: "THE MANLY THING TONIC"

This is the man's man tonic. Many of the same ingredients were used in what was known as the "root" tonic in the Wild West. It seems that cowboys were really into being manly and strong, and these items were brewed together to help them stay that way. All of the ingredients have the reputation of being body strengtheners as well as sex-drive boosters. Some might even call them aphrodisiacs. Remember: healthy bodies have healthy sex drives.

4 cups dates
½ cup saw palmetto berries
½ cup ginger
¼ cup sarsaparilla
¼ cup licorice
¼ cup ginseng
¼ cup astragalus
1 gallon water

Place all the ingredients in a covered pot and heat them on medium for 30 minutes. The ingredients should be at a low boil the entire time. Stir constantly. After the allotted cooking time, strain the mixture, bottle it, and refrigerate. The cowboys took a swig of this every day to keep all parts involved riding high in the saddle.

FOR THE GIRLS:
"THE WOMANLY THING TONIC"

This is the woman's tonic supreme, concocted from herbs used around the world for centuries to strengthen the female constitution. The active ingredient is angelica. The Chinese say that the daily intake of angelica will keep women "beautiful" well beyond the usual expiration date. Rather than seeing this as a sexist statement, I think of it is a health statement. Isn't beauty, masculine and feminine, indicative of vigor and vitality?

½ cup angelica
½ cup astragalus
½ cup licorice
½ cup mint
2 tablespoons freshly ground ginger
2 tablespoons lemon balm
2 tablespoons cinnamon
1 gallon water
4 cups honey

Place all the ingredients except the honey in a covered pot and boil for 30 minutes. Strain the mixture, cool the liquid, add honey, bottle the mixture, and store it in the refrigerator. As with most tonics, a tablespoon a day is said to keep the doctor away.

"ONE TOO MANY
LAST NIGHT TONIC"

Though I don't drink alcohol and recommend that everybody lay off the sauce, billboards coast to coast indicate drinking is the United States' national pastime. This means that liver damaging is the national sport. If you drink enough to feel the effect of alcohol, you are damaging your liver and should consider taking better care of it. In fact, some herbalists feel that the amount of toxins in our environment and in our food supply indicate that we should all be taking a liver tonic on a daily basis.

1 cup dandelion root or leaves
2 teaspoons blessed thistle
2 teaspoons burdock
2 teaspoons yellow dock
2 teaspoons ginseng
2 teaspoons astragalus
2 teaspoons lemon balm
2 teaspoons mint
1 gallon water
2 cups honey

Heat water to boiling and add all the ingredients except the honey. Allow the mixture to boil 5 minutes, turn off the heat, and let the pot cool. Strain, add honey, and store in the refrigerator. If I've been in a toxic situation, like a junk-food binge, I will take a cup or two a day for a week to help my body clean out all the nasty chemicals. This is an especially good beverage during the holiday season.

"WHAT YOU GOT, I DON'T WANT TONIC"

As I pass through life, I come into contact with lots of people, and it's shocking how many head into populated places fully knowing that they have infectious diseases. Folks think they are doing the world a favor, coming into the office when they're sick. Many times I've sat next to coughing, hacking, choking beings, and this thought always comes to mind: "What you got, I don't want." Whenever I feel I've been exposed to something and I want to help my body fight its takeover, I pull this tonic out of the refrigerator, pour myself a shot, and keep doing this for several days. All of the ingredients are mildly antibiotic and have long histories of use in treating breakouts of infectious diseases.

Take all of the ingredients except the honey and boil them until the liquid has reduced by half and the dates have thoroughly dissolved. While the mixture is boiling, stir constantly. When the solution is cool, strain it to remove the herbs and date skins, add honey, mix well, bottle it, and store it in the refrigerator. Take a cup a day for a week after you've been exposed to something nasty.

4 cups dates
¼ cup angelica
¼ cup astragalus
¼ cup burdock
¼ cup blessed thistle
¼ cup echinacea
¼ cup ginger
¼ cup licorice
¼ cup lemon balm
¼ cup red clover
1 gallon water
4 cups honey

"THE PRETTY PARLOR TONIC"

There is only one thing nicer than having other people treat you right, and that's treating yourself right. This tonic is part of a treatment that I call "The Pretty Parlor." First take a handful each of lavender, mint, lemon balm, myrrh, and rosemary, toss them into a gallon of boiling water, and pour the whole kit and caboodle into a tub of hot water. Dive in, soak as long as you like, and when you step out of the tub, rub yourself down with this lotion made of skin-healing herbs (or let someone else do the job). It can be used for an overall body treatment or to rub on a patch of sore skin—take your pick.

1 cup angelica
1 cup burdock
1 cup dandelion root or leaves
1 cup lemon balm
1 cup mint
1 cup plantain
1 cup red clover
1 cup Saint-John's-wort
1 cup self-heal prunella
4 tablespoons honey
2 cups olive oil
1 cup cocoa butter
1 cup sesame oil
1 cup vodka
1 cup hot water

Grind all the herbs in a food processor or pulverize them by hand. Place ground herbs in a large salad bowl and cover them with the oils, vodka, and hot water. Cover well and let sit in a cool location for one month. Then pour the mixture into the leg of a new pair of pantyhose, collecting the liquid in a clean pot. When the pantyhose leg has stopped dripping, put the liquid in a bottle. Shake well before using. This can be stored in the open indefinitely—the alcohol keeps it fresh.

"WILL THIS COLD EVER GO AWAY? TONIC"

I use this formula whenever I get a cold that won't move on. All of the ingredients are respiratory strengtheners with mild antibiotic effects. The combination has helped me kick out many a nasty cold that would have otherwise hung on for dear life.

4 lemons
½ cup astragalus
½ cup burdock
½ cup echinacea
1 cup ginger
1 cup licorice
½ cup Saint-John's-wort
1 cup mint
1 clove garlic
1 gallon water
2 cups honey

Juice the lemons, retaining both juice and rinds. Add all the ingredients to a pot, including the lemon rinds but minus the juice and honey, cover, and boil until the water has reduced by half. Strain and add honey and lemon juice to the remaining liquid. I take a tablespoon every four hours until three days after the cold has passed.

"GUT-ROT TONIC NUMBER TWO"

People underestimate the importance of the stomach. In fact, many take their stomachs for granted, and that's a big mistake. Like the liver, the stomach is a body part you always want to keep in fine shape. Rather than abusing it, I think we all should revere it, and taking this tonic is one way to do that. The following ingredients are all classics used to tonify the stomach, relax it, and keep it running smoothly.

3 cups mint
1 cup angelica
1 cup garlic
½ cup cinnamon
½ cup ginger
½ cup lemon balm
2 quarts water
2 cups honey

Add all the ingredients except the honey, bring them to a rolling boil, and reduce the liquid down to two cups. Strain the mixture and add honey to the liquid. I keep this tonic in the refrigerator and take a teaspoon now and then. People who have frequent stomach complaints might want to take a good look at what they are doing to and for their stomachs.

GETTING YOUR HERBS

W hether you are planning to make my "Turbo Tonic" or one of the more specific tonics, you are going to need a ready supply of the 30 life-saving plants. You have several options: you can grow your own, buy the herbs at a natural food store or herb shop, order them through the mail, or gather them from the wild.

GROWING YOUR OWN

My favorite part of making homemade tonics is running out to the backyard and gathering up a big handful of disease-preventing plants. There is something really wonderful about having tonic plants thriving in my backyard, waiting for me to use them. Many of the 30 top tonic plants are extremely simple to grow. In fact, most of them are so easy that it's a crime to pay money for them.

With readers all over the globe, I will not even attempt to give specific instructions for all the possible growing sites. Not only is it a waste of space, it's also beyond the scope of this book. Don't despair, though, the information you need is easy enough to obtain.

If you want to plant some of these herbs, and I heartily suggest that you do so, your best sources for instructions are herb-growing books and herb growers. The books can be found at any library; the herb growers, who are perhaps your best source, are usually a phone call or a letter away.

For anyone interested in growing herbs, there exists an invaluable institution which is otherwise known as the mail-order herb nursery. These companies are accustomed to shipping their wares around the world, and as such, they are in contact with herb growers everywhere. Their staffs know their plants and can give you lots of helpful information about growing specific herbs in your specific region.

I have been gardening for some time, and I will be the first to agree that most books don't answer the weird little questions you have. This is largely due to space constraints. It does not mean that you don't need the questions answered, it means that books are limited.

I have found that mail-order growers are both interested and kind enough to answer any and all of your questions. So rather than trying to give you instructions, I will give you the names of some mail-order companies from which you can get both your herbs and your herb-growing information. Here's the list:

Companion Plants
7247 N. Coolville Ridge Road
Athens, OH 45701
(614) 592-4643

Dabney Herb Farm
Box 22061
Louisville, KY 40222
(502) 893-5198

Fox Hill Farm
444 W. Michigan Avenue, Box 9
Parma, MI 49269
(517) 531-3179

The Herb Cottage
(seeds only)
Washington Cathedral
Mt. St. Alban
Washington, DC 20016
(202) 537-8982

Rasland Farm
N.C. 82 at U.S. 13
Godwin, NC 28344
(919) 567-2705

The Rosemary House
120 S. Market Street
Mechanicsburg, PA 17055
(717) 697-5111 or (717) 766-6581

Sandy Mush Herb Nursery
Rt. 2, Surrett Cove Road
Leicester, NC 28748
(704) 683-2014

Taylor's Herb Garden
1535 Lone Oak Road
Vista, CA 92084
(619) 727-3485

Triple Oaks Nursery and Florist
Franklinville, NJ 08322
(609) 694-4272

Village Arbors
1804 Saugahatchee Road
Alburn, AL 36830
(205) 826-3490
(800) 288-5033

Well-Sweep Herb Farm
317 Mt. Bethel Road
Port Murray, NJ 07865
(908) 852-5390

Wyrttun Ward
Beach Street RFD
Middleboro, MA 02346
(617) 866-4087

If you are growing your own herbs, you will have to collect them to use them. This is what we call harvesting, and it's quite simple: go out and grab what you want. I find that the best time to make tonics is midsummer when many of the plants are at their largest and most abundant. Being a bit lazy, I would rather use the few plants that aren't quite at their peak at a less-than-ideal moment than go through the process of drying and storing them for later use.

However, if you want to harvest each one at the height of its perfection, here is a chart which may be of use to you:

Plant	Part Used	Best Time to Collect
Angelica	Root	Fall
Barberry	Berries, Root	Summer
Blessed Thistle	Whole plant	When in bloom
Burdock	Root	Fall
Astragalus	Root	Fall
Dandelion	Root, Leaves	Fall
Echinacea	Whole plant	Fall
Figs	Fruit	Summer
Garlic	Bulb	When leaves die back
Ginseng	Root	Fall
Grape	Fruit	Summer
Jujube	Fruit	Summer
Juniper	Fruit	Early fall
Lemon Balm	Leaves, Stems	Early summer
Licorice	Root	Fall
Mint	Leaves, Stems	Early summer
Mustard	Seed, Leaves	Spring, Summer
Plantain	Whole plant	Year around
Red Clover	Flower, Plant	June
Saint-John's-wort	Whole plant	When in bloom
Sarsaparilla	Root	Fall
Saw Palmetto	Fruit	Summer
Schizandra	Fruit	Summer
Self-heal Prunella	Whole plant	Year around
Yellow Dock	Root	Fall

Clip them or dig them up (depending on what part you are harvesting), shake any bugs or dirt from them, and spread them out in a dry, sunless area. The space needs to have air circulation, but no direct light, which would destroy the plants' essential oils. When they are crispy dry, which should take about two days, store them in zip-lock bags.

GETTING HERBS LOCALLY

If you live in or around a major city, there is bound to be a decent herb seller somewhere nearby. Look in the Yellow Pages and call around until you find someone who sells "loose" herbs. Some stores sell prepackaged herbs, which tend to be much more expensive than herbs sold loose because you're paying for packaging you don't need. Herb stores that sell loose herbs usually do a large enough volume that you can reasonably assume the stuff is fresh. It's something that's not often brought up about packaged herbs, but they can sit around on the shelf for a long, long time, losing their potency all the while.

ORDERING DRIED HERBS THROUGH THE MAIL

There are a number of reputable, and I stress the word reputable, dealers in dried herbs who will ship whatever it is you want right to your front door. You send for a catalogue, fill out the order form, and—zoom, zoom—your ingredients are in a box in the kitchen. It couldn't be easier:

Aphrodisia
264 Bleecker Street
New York, NY 10014
(212) 989-6440

Blessed Herbs
Michael Volchok
Rt. 5, Box 1042
Ava, MO 65608
(417) 683-5721

Brion Corporation
1945 Palo Verde Avenue
Long Beach, CA 90716
(310) 493-5405
(for Chinese herb formulas and extracts)

Circle Sanctuary Herbs
P. O. Box 219
Mt. Horeb, WI 53572
(608) 924-2216

Dr. Michael's Herb Center
5109 Northwestern Avenue
Chicago, IL 60625
(312) 271-7738

Essence of Life Ministries
Mike and Debby Minear, herbalists
Rt. 1, Box 172
Little Hocking, OH 45742
(614) 989-2300

Great China Herb Company
857 Washington Street
San Francisco, CA 94108
(415) 982-2195

The Herb and Spice Collection
Box 118
Norway, IA 52318
(800) 786-1388

Herb-Pharm
(liquid extracts only)
P. O. Box 116
Williams, OR 97544

Island Herbs
Ryan Drum
Waldron Island, WA 98297

Meadowbrook Herb Garden
Route 138
Wyoming, RI 02898
(401) 539-7603

Meer Corporation
9500 Railroad Avenue
N. Bergen, NJ 07047
(201) 861-9500

Reevis Mountain School of Survival
2025 North Third Street
Phoenix, AZ 85004
(602) 252-6019

Tai Sang Trading Chinese Herb Company
1018 Stockton Street
San Francisco, CA 94108
(415) 981-5364

Trinity Herb
P. O. Box 199
Bodega, CA 94922
(707) 874-3418

Trout Lake Herb Farm
149 Little Mountain Road
Trout Lake, WA 98650
(509) 395-2025

COLLECTING YOUR OWN FROM THE WILD

Your last option is to go out and collect the herbs that grow wild in and around civilization. These are:

Angelica
Barberry
Burdock
Dandelion
Echinacea
Ginseng
Grape
Mustard
Plantain
Red Clover
Saint-John's-wort
Sarsaparilla
Self-heal Prunella
Yellow Dock

If you are not familiar with these plants, use a field guide for positive identification. If you can't positively identify the plant, don't use it! Also, don't pick herbs that are likely to have been sprayed with chemicals, as this defeats the purpose. If you are foolish enough to have your lawn sprayed by a chemical company, don't use the dandelions growing in it. Remember, these outfits put down tons and tons of "insecticides." Toxin-filled dandelions won't do your liver any favors.

It is best to use these herbs immediately after collecting them. You can dry them for later use, but as always, the rule of thumb is: the fresher, the better.

A CLOSING NOTE:

I have given you some of my favorite recipes, and they are just that, *my* favorite recipes. You may like them as they stand, or you may want to improve upon them. In the old days, everyone made tonics, and everybody had his or her own favorite recipe. Folks experimented, adding a little of this or that until in time they came up with a tonic combination they believed in. So feel free to take the information and recipes I have given you and play around with them.

You may want to create your own special-needs tonic. Figure out what physical weaknesses you have and research the tonic plants that will strengthen these deficiencies. What I have provided in this book is only a tiny sampling of all the information that's out there. Go ahead, dive in, formulate a tonic tailor-made to keep *you* well, and by all means have fun in the process!

162
quarta